The Natural Way

Allergies

Moira Crawford

Series medical consultants
Dr Peter Albright MD (USA)
& Dr David Peters MD (UK)

Approved by the
AMERICAN HOLISTIC MEDICAL ASSOCIATION &
BRITISH HOLISTIC MEDICAL ASSOCIATION

KT-378-813

ELEMENT
Shaftesbury, Dorset • Boston, Massachusetts
Melbourne, Victoria

© Element Books Limited 1997
Text © Moira Crawford 1997

First published in the UK in 1997 by
Element Books Limited
Shaftesbury, Dorset, SP7 8BP

Published in the USA in 1997 by
Element Books, Inc.
160 North Washington St, Boston MA 02114

Published in Australia in 1997 by
Element Books and distributed by
Penguin Books Australia Limited
487 Maroondah Highway
Ringwood, Victoria 3134

Cover design by Slatter-Anderson
Text illustrations by David Gifford
Designed and typeset by Intype
Printed and bound in Great Britain by
Caledonian International Book Manufacturers, Glasgow

British Library Cataloguing in Publication data available

Library of Congress Cataloging in Publication data

ISBN 1 86204 114 8

Contents

Illustrations   v
Introduction   vii

Chapter 1   **What is allergy?**   1
Chapter 2   **How allergy affects people**   12
Chapter 3   **Causes and trigger factors**   20
Chapter 4   **How to help yourself**   31
Chapter 5   **Conventional medical treatment**   45
Chapter 6   **The natural therapies and allergy**   56
Chapter 7   **Treating the body**   66
Chapter 8   **Treating the mind and emotions**   92
Chapter 9   **Diet and nutritional therapy**   104
Chapter 10 **How to find and choose a practitioner**   115

Appendix A **Glossary of words connected with
                allergy and intolerance**   124
Appendix B **Useful addresses**   126
Appendix C **Useful further reading**   130
Index   132

Illustrations

Figure 1   The acupuncture 'energy' meridians   70
Figure 2   Craniosacral techniques   82
Figure 3   Reflex zones on the right foot   88
Figure 4   The Lotus position   102

Introduction

It is estimated that around 10 per cent of people who seek medical help do so because of problems caused by allergies or intolerances. This figure is likely to rise even further over the coming years due to the ever-increasing variety of substances to which we are exposed and to which human beings can become sensitized. Allergy is a classic 'disease of civilization' – to make our lives more comfortable we have developed ever more substances to which our bodies may react. These range from industrial pollution to cars and the foods and chemicals we use in our homes. Additionally, the last 50 years have seen our diet change beyond all recognition. Previous generations ate the same foods as their grandparents and great-grandparents had eaten; now, with convenience foods, ice cream and other imported and manufactured dishes, our bodies have had to learn very quickly to process completely different types of food. It is not surprising that sometimes our bodies cannot cope. Modern living also builds stress – many people find that otherwise controlled allergies or intolerance may break out when they are under pressure.

Allergy affects different people in different ways, from the relatively straightforward symptoms of hayfever which come on following a walk in the park on a sunny day – a true allergy – to a number of vaguer symptoms for which it is difficult to trace a common cause, which are often described as an intolerance. For those with multiple allergies or intolerances, the condition can be debilitating and impose significant restrictions on their way of life. The effects are often emotional and psychological, as well as physical – many people with allergies or intolerances become anxious or depressed as well as suffering from their allergic or intolerant symptoms.

Conventional medicine has produced many effective treatments for allergy, but these tend to concentrate simply on the management of the symptoms, without treating the underlying cause. If the treatment is stopped, the allergy may return – maybe even more severely.

Complementary practitioners tend to see allergies and intolerances in a wider context – as external signs of underlying imbalance or deficiency in the body. Different approaches to diet, or physical therapies such as acupuncture, homeopathy or osteopathy, aim to correct the imbalances, strengthening the body and enabling it to start the process of self-healing. Therapies that address the mind and emotions, such as meditation or visualization, help the sufferer to reverse the downward emotional spiral and begin to take a positive attitude to life again, in turn improving his or her own well-being.

In allergy, perhaps more than in most conditions, the sufferer is the one best placed to help him- or herself, and there is a great deal that you can do to identify your own trigger factors, reduce your exposure to them, and improve your own health. The aim of this book is to give you the information and the tools to start to heal yourself and to know where to go if you need help. If you put yourself in charge, you will be well on the way to solving the problem.

Moira Crawford
Suffolk 1997

CHAPTER 1

What is allergy?

Snoopy famously once said: 'I'm allergic to mornings.'
We all know what he meant. We've heard people claim
to be 'allergic' to everything from pollen, eggs and
seafood to washing powder, and we know that they
mean that a particular food or substance doesn't agree
with them. In fact, the term allergy is often taken now to
mean almost anything from a life-threatening condition,
such as the severe reaction some people have had to
peanuts, to a simple intense dislike of a food or product.

Over the last 30 years, there has been a dramatic
increase in the amount of 'allergic' disease reported
worldwide and the epidemic is gathering speed. Because
allergy takes many forms, it is impossible to specify a
strict set of symptoms. However, asthma, eczema, hay
fever and hives, or urticaria, are commonly caused by
allergies or intolerances either to foods or to substances
breathed in with the air or which touch our skin. All
are on the increase, especially in the industrialized or
developed parts of the world.

In the United States, some doctors claim that up to
60 per cent of the population suffer from symptoms
associated with food intolerances, with around 7 per cent
suffering from eczema. In the Western world, up to 30
per cent of the population have an allergic tendency –
that is, they are prone to developing an allergy – and
probably one in four people will suffer from an allergy

at some time in their life. By contrast, however, in less developed countries, asthma and hay fever are almost unknown. Research is pointing ever more convincingly to the fact that the environment that we have created is contributing more and more to our ill-health. Figures from the US National Heart, Lung and Blood Institute suggest that around 12.4 million Americans suffer from asthma – almost double the figure of 6.8 million in the 1980s. Over 4 million of these sufferers are under 18 years of age.

Anyone can become allergic – to almost anything – and the degree of severity of the allergy can range from a minor inconvenience to a major health hazard. People who are allergic to caviar, for example, will not find avoiding it a great restriction of their freedom, but someone with an extreme allergy to common foods such as eggs or dairy products must be very careful with food prepared by another person, as they are often hidden in cakes, sauces and other dishes. A woman with a violent reaction to rubber was reported recently in a UK women's magazine as living in constant anxiety from the hidden threat to her health from rubber bands, elastic, rubber foam-filled seats, bath mats, hosepipes and even in the possibility of her inhaling particles of rubber from car tyres in busy streets. Her allergy, combined with the anxiety it has caused her, has resulted in the loss of her job in an office and a seriously restricted lifestyle.

Defining allergies

An allergy occurs when the body becomes over-sensitive to something – a food or another substance – and the immune system overreacts every time it comes into contact with it. That is, it is an exaggerated defensive reaction by the body's immune system to an otherwise harmless substance. In order to understand this process, we need first to explain the role of the immune system, and how it becomes involved in an allergic reaction (*see box*).

The immune system and allergy

The immune system is the body's defence mechanism and is vital to protect us from infections. When an external organism, such as a virus or bacteria, enters the body, the immune system springs into action with a range of defences to fight off infection. Swelling, redness and fever are all typical signs of a battle taking place between the defences of the immune system and the outsider, known as an antigen, and are a healthy indication that the immune system is in working order. In allergy, however, the immune system is hypersensitive. It overreacts to an otherwise harmless substance, such as dust, pollen or a foodstuff. It may take one or many exposures for the allergy to develop, but the system mistakes a harmless substance for an enemy, or allergen, and sends lymphocytes, a type of white blood cell, to the rescue. These create antibodies to fight the invader. Once the first contact has been made, one type of lymphocyte, known as the B cell, memorizes the allergen, so that it can create antibodies quickly should it return. This is known as sensitization, and means that the allergy sufferer from then on will react to that substance whenever he or she comes into contact with it again. The antibody most commonly created in allergy is known as immunoglobulin E, or IgE. This attaches itself to mast cells, located in the skin, the nose, mouth, throat and gastrointestinal tract, and basophils (white cells) in the bloodstream. When the allergen appears again, the IgE acts to activate the mast cells and trigger the release of chemicals, in particular histamine, which causes immediate symptoms such as sneezing, sore and runny eyes, rashes, tingling, vomiting or diarrhoea, depending on the allergen and the sufferer's individual reaction.

Atopic individuals, who have a genetic or inherited disposition towards allergy (*see* page 9 have been found to have higher than normal levels of IgE in their bodies, making them more disposed than others towards allergic reactions of any sort.

The commonest allergens

Pollen and moulds
Insect stings
Some foods, especially eggs, dairy products, fish and nuts, citrus fruits, certain cereals, coffee
House dust mite droppings
Fur or dander (skin scales) from pets
Some chemicals in the home or work environment
Some medicines (eg, penicillin, aspirin)

The response to an allergy is usually immediate. In hay fever or allergic asthma, for example, the reaction comes on within seconds after exposure to the allergen. Allergies tend to affect the skin, respiratory (breathing) system or gastrointestinal system. In a typical hay fever reaction, for example, the immune system acts to release histamine, causing the typical symptoms of runny nose and eyes, sneezing, irritation and itch.

There are two main types of skin reaction in allergy. Eczema due to an allergy (also called atopic dermatitis) occurs in those people who produce an excess of immunoglobulin E (IgE), making them liable to become sensitive to a number of allergens. Eczema can cause extremely itchy dry skin and the condition is becoming more common, particularly among children, but fortunately many grow out of it.

Contact eczema, more common in adults, is caused by a specific allergy developed through touching a certain substance or subtances.

A second type of skin reaction, with many possible causes, is urticaria, also known as nettlerash or hives. This may last from a few hours to several days. With a classic food allergy the reaction may often be quick, including vomiting, diarrhoea and abdominal (stomach) pain.

An extreme of this type of allergic reaction is anaphylaxis, a generalized allergic reaction which gets out of control and affects the entire body. This can be fatal if it is not treated appropriately and immediately (*see box*). Peanut allergy, for example, now claims several lives in the USA each year.

Anaphylaxis

In an extreme allergic reaction, anaphylaxis can occur. This potentially fatal condition affects the entire body and can occur in minutes if the sufferer is extremely sensitive. Nuts, particularly peanuts, have featured in recent headlines about deaths due to anaphylaxis, but other foods can cause it, as can reactions to drugs and insect stings. Symptoms include severe urticaria (rash) all over the body, swelling of the throat, breathing difficulty, nausea, vomiting, a sudden drop in blood pressure and loss of consciousness. Anaphylaxis is a life-threatening condition which requires immediate medical attention and injected adrenaline.

These types of allergy often come on in childhood and young adulthood, and may settle as the sufferer gets older. They are usually fairly easy to identify, as the reaction is close to the trigger.

Symptoms of allergies

Respiratory: hay fever, rhinitis, asthma
Eyes: conjunctivitis
Skin: rash, itching, swelling (oedema)
Gastrointestinal: vomiting, abdominal pain, diarrhoea
General (in extreme cases): anaphylaxis (swelling of
mucous membranes and constriction of breathing, allergic
shock)

Defining intolerances

By definition, an allergy involves an immune response to
the allergen, but other reactions, particularly to foods, are
known as pseudo-allergies, sensitivities or intolerances.

Some foods trigger reactions or contain substances that
harm the body in some way. Coeliac disease, an intolerance of the protein gluten found in wheat, rye, barley
and some other cereals, is thought to be caused by the
food damaging the lining of the intestine, and preventing
the natural absorption of nutrients. It may be that a
food contains a certain chemical that affects you, such as
histamine, found in fermented foods such as cheese, or certain fish. Here the histamine acts directly on the body,
rather than being created by it as in an allergic reaction.

Caffeine, found in coffee, colas, tea, chocolate and
some painkillers, works on the nervous system,
and affects some people more adversely than others.

Hyperactivity in children may be caused by an intolerance to certain additives in foods. The yellow food dye,
tartrazine, has most frequently been found to cause intolerance as well as behavioural problems.

Sometimes the problem is caused by a defect in the
individual – some people are deficient in the necessary
enzymes to break down certain foods. For example, a

deficiency of lactase, which is necessary for digesting milk and milk products, causes milk intolerance.

Sensitivities to other substances, such as detergents, chemicals or dust in the working environment, may be caused by their concentration – the skin or the airways may simply be irritated by over-exposure to them.

Increasingly, the 'leaky gut syndrome' is becoming accepted and recognized as a possible cause of food intolerances (*see box*).

Leaky gut syndrome

Leaky gut syndrome is a problem identified by many nutritionists as responsible for a large number of problems, such as certain forms of arthritis, which initially may not be put down to an allergy or intolerance. As its name suggests, the lining of the bowel becomes irritated, for example due to an allergy or the overuse of antibiotics, and becomes permeable. As a result, partially digested proteins escape into the bloodstream. It can be difficult for the body to break down these proteins and if some of them are similar to the proteins which occur naturally in the body, they can act as chemical triggers which, for instance, produce muscle contraction in blood vessels (causing migraine, for example) or in the intestine itself (causing irritable bowel). Furthermore – and this is not proven by research – although many complementary practitioners believe it to be so, if the proteins cannot be eliminated in the usual way (through urine or faeces) they may appear in other organs and lead to inflammation. This occurs particularly in the joints and skin, and at weak points, and naturopaths and nutritional therapists suspect that sometimes it causes 'allergic arthritis'. Dietary therapy and the use of probiotics which allow the bowel to heal, can have dramatic results.

Intolerances are much more difficult to diagnose than allergies. Allergies can be detected simply by skin or blood tests which show the involvement of the immune system. Tests for the causes of intolerances, however, are less conclusive and remain controversial in the eyes of scientific medicine.

Intolerances are usually not immediately linked to exposure to the allergen; in fact, they are often caused by a substance with which the sufferer is in constant daily contact. Symptoms may often seem to bear no relation to one another and, in the case of mood swings, anxiety or forgetfulness, may appear to be more psychological than physical. What's more, there are an increasing number of illnesses, such as chronic fatigue syndrome and irritable bowel syndrome, which have chronic, apparently unrelated symptoms. Some practitioners have found that these conditions may be due to intolerances.

Symptoms of intolerances

A huge range of symptoms may be caused by an intolerance. The following most commonly experienced symptoms show how difficult it is to pin them down to a biochemical reason. Many of the symptoms are psychological and it may be that a problem is as much 'holistic' as 'cellular' – that is, it concerns a person's whole self – mind, body and spirit – not just one part of them. However, such reactions may play a part in causing:

Fatigue and lethargy
Mood swings
Food cravings (see 'masking')
Sleep disturbance and insomnia
Depression or anxiety
Lack of concentration

Dizziness
Memory failure
Weight gain
Swelling of joints
Aches and pains
Headaches and migraines
Hayfever
Sneezing
Itches
Eczema
Dry skin
Hair loss
Asthma
Wheezing, cough, frequent 'colds'
Recurring urticaria
Thrush (candidiasis)
Cystitis
Constipation and/or diarrhoea
Bloating, wind and stomach pain
Mouth ulcers

Who gets allergies or intolerances?

There are no rules on who can and cannot develop an allergy or intolerance, but certain people are at higher risk. A major factor in the development of true allergic disease is a genetic or inherited predisposition towards allergy, known as 'atopy'. Atopy is a family tendency which increases the risk that a person will develop one or more allergies. If one parent is atopic, a child has around a 30 per cent likelihood of being atopic too; if both parents are atopic, the risk rises to over 60 per cent. Several allergies are linked – for example, within a family it is not uncommon for different members to suffer from eczema, asthma and hay fever, or all three. Many atopic people who are suffering from a food allergy or intolerance find that they react to more than one type of food and, again, that family members suffer in a similar way. The brothers and sisters of atopic children are especially likely to develop an allergic tendency. Atopy is seen in three very common instances:

- atopic dermatitis (eczema)
- hay fever (rhinitis, symptoms which involve the nose, and conjunctivitis, sore eyes)
- allergic asthma.

Allergies may also 'skip' a generation, so a child may inherit his or her grandparents' tendency to allergy. Boys appear to be more disposed towards developing atopic asthma, although the sex difference is not pronounced in other allergic conditions.

Other factors appear to influence a person's predisposition to allergy, especially low birth weight. Small and premature babies seem particularly prone to allergies; it is thought because their immune system is not developed enough to prevent sensitivities from developing. The season of birth appears to make a difference, too. Winter babies, have a noticeably lower tendency to allergy, particularly asthma, probably because the concentrations of allergens are lower at the time just after birth when they are most vulnerable.

Smoking can also be a culprit for causing allergies. Smoking by a mother before birth and exposure to passive smoking after birth raise the chances of allergy in a child. Occupational allergic disease is growing in prevalence. It occurs when someone becomes sensitized to a substance they come into contact with at work, often a particle in the air such as dust or flour, or a chemical or other substance with which they work. Increasingly, health professionals are discovering that they have become sensitized to their latex gloves. Furthermore, hairdressers are becoming sensitized to the dyes, shampoos and other substances which they handle constantly.

Allergies and infants

Allergies in babies and small children, which are rising in incidence, can be particularly distressing and frightening for parents. Asthma attacks can be life-threatening and immediate medical attention should be sought, as it should for any extreme reaction, particularly a swelling of the mouth which may indicate the start of an anaphylactic reaction.

Eczema is itchy and distressing for the child, and for the parents trying to prevent their offspring from scratching themselves raw. Chapter 4 gives some practical tips on coping which this problem. Aside from drugs and soothing agents, gentle alternatives are available which aim to address the underlying cause of the allergy. Particularly effective in dealing with both physical problems and emotional difficulties in infants on a non-verbal level, are cranial osteopathy and craniosacral therapy (*see* pages 82–5). Babies only a few months old can also benefit from the careful use of Chinese herbs, made up in compresses, creams and lotions. It is important that you consult a qualified practitioner.

Whatever the cause of your own or your child's allergy or intolerance, however, the first step is to identify it. The following chapters will discuss the symptoms of the different types of allergy and intolerance, and will try to give you pointers so that you can identify them, test for them, avoid them, treat your symptoms and, we hope, solve the underlying problem. With patience and the right approach for you, the long-term aim is to strengthen your own system so that it can heal its own problems. In the meantime, however, the first goal will be to put you, not your allergy, in charge of your life.

CHAPTER 2

How allergy affects people

Allergy affects different people in different ways, which is why the problem is so difficult to define, diagnose and treat. It was thought that the reaction was 'at the point of entry' so that inhaled allergens caused the respiratory (breathing) and eye problems of asthma and hay fever, and food allergies or intolerances caused vomiting, diarrhoea and other gastrointestinal problems. Likewise, touching or wearing a substance to which a person was allergic would be expected to cause swelling or a rash at the site.

But it is not that simple. It has been shown now that food allergies and intolerances can cause skin reactions and respiratory problems, and that physical contact with certain substances can also cause respiratory problems. Allergies or intolerances which involve a number of apparently random symptoms may sometimes be caused by all types of allergens, alone and in combination, so the picture can be very confusing.

Hayfever

Hayfever, properly called allergic rhinitis, is a classic example of an acute reaction, and is commonly experienced by atopic people. The condition is on the increase and is nowadays particularly severe in built-up areas, where pollution and fumes reduce the air quality and cause increasing amounts of allergy.

In hay fever, when the allergen is inhaled, the immune system recognizes an enemy and activates the mast cells to release the chemical mediators, particularly histamine. This causes a 'cascade' effect, involving sneezing and a watery discharge from the nose. The nose and sometimes the roof of the mouth become itchy, a feeling that can spread into the throat and towards the ears. If the hay fever sufferer comes into contact with a particularly strong concentration of the allergen – for example, on days of especially poor air quality or a very high pollen count – the nose may become blocked and the discharge thick. Many hay fever sufferers experience headaches and general malaise (feeling under par). As the condition is most common in the summer months when the weather is fine, it is an especially cruel blow as hay fever sufferers need to stay indoors to avoid inducing the symptoms.

Perennial rhinitis is a kind of year-round hay fever, which involves the same reactions, but can be triggered by substances not related to the seasons – for example, the house dust mite (*see* Chapter 3).

Allergic conjunctivitis

Allergic conjunctivitis, often called 'hay fever eyes', is an eye condition related to hay fever. In allergic conjunctivitis, once the immune system has been primed (sensitized) IgE sticks on to the surface of mast cells in the mucous membrane lining the eyes. When the allergen is encountered again, the allergic reaction is set off, and certain chemicals, including histamine, prostaglandins and cytokines are released. The effects of this include a swelling of the bood vessels and irritation of the nerve endings in the eye. This results in the typical 'red eye' of allergic conjunctivitis. The eye can be puffy and is often very itchy – a feature made worse by rubbing. It also tends to water. Normally both eyes are affected, but the condition can be one-sided – for example, if a cat hair is accidentally rubbed into one eye.

Allergic asthma

There are several types of asthma, not all related to allergy, but atopic or allergic asthma affects people with sensitive respiratory systems. Bronchial hypersensitivity may be due to a number of factors, including pollen, dust, cigarette smoke or exhaust fumes, and chemical or household fumes, such as air fresheners. Allergy is thought to underlie the development of this hypersensitivity in 80–90 per cent of children and in 50–60 per cent of adults with asthma by causing inflammation in the airways. In an attack, the asthma sufferer's bronchi, or airways, tighten up due to a spasm (involuntary contractions of the muscles), oedema (swelling of the mucous membrane in the bronchi), and an excessive production of mucus. The net result is that they find difficulty in breathing, especially in exhaling. This is a very frightening experience which, if it is not treated promptly, can be life-threatening.

Occupational asthma is a condition caused by sensitization to a substance inhaled at the workplace. The asthma tends to get worse at work and for a while after leaving, but the condition improves at weekends or holidays. The symptoms are much like those of atopic (allergic) asthma, but tend to be cyclical, improving and worsening as the sufferer is exposed to the allergen at work. It is believed that around 5 per cent of asthma is due to occupational asthma. Professions that are affected include workers in sawmills or grain and flour mills, and farmers and laboratory workers, but anyone breathing in dust or other particles at work could be at risk.

Eczema

Like asthma, eczema can be due to a number of causes, but it is often associated with allergy. It is particularly common among children of atopic families who have high levels of immunoglobulin E (IgE), making them susceptible to a number of allergens.

Atopic eczema usually starts before the age of two, and often in the first few months of life. Between 5 per cent and 15 per cent of schoolchildren are estimated to have atopic eczema, but fortunately the condition often improves as the child gets older. It can come on, however, during the teenage years or in young adulthood. People who have suffered from atopic eczema as children will probably find that even if the eczema clears, they will always have a tendency towards dry, scaly skin. As the cause is effectively an internal disorder, pressures on the system, such as stress, play a major role in causing outbreaks of eczema in atopic people. The problem may remain under control for most of the time, but, when stress levels get too high, an attack of eczema may result.

Food allergies or intolerances may be to blame, and often already dry skin can break out into eczema after the classic allergenic foods such as dairy products or eggs have been eaten. Processed food is a particular culprit, as additives within it may be well concealed.

Inhaled substances can cause or certainly exacerbate eczema. Many sufferers from atopic eczema will find that the condition is made worse by contact with pets or birds, and that it may be more severe in the summer months when they are also likely to be suffering from hay fever.

Atopic eczema sufferers are, of course, particularly

likely to suffer from allergies to substances they touch, wear or handle in the course of their work. These are discussed in more detail under 'contact allergies' (*see* Chapter 3).

Eczema is particularly distressing for both the child suffering from it and the parents, as the itching is unbearable and children may have to be restrained to stop them scratching and making the condition worse. The sufferer's skin becomes dry and itchy, especially at night, and the action of scratching releases histamine from the skin, increasing the itch, and making it red and inflamed. If the sufferer continues to scratch, the eczema can bleed and become infected and weepy.

Eczema can occur on any part of the body, although in babies it usually starts on the face, scalp and diaper area. Flexures (behind the knees and inside the elbows and wrists) are common spots for eczema to appear in toddlers and older children. In particularly severe and distressing cases, however, the eczema can spread all over the body.

Another type of eczema related to allergy is contact eczema, caused by increased exposure to irritants, rather than being due to the internal mechanism of atopy. This is particularly related to an allergy to a specific substance, such as nickel, rubber, cosmetics, chemicals such as household or DIY products, and, quite commonly, sticking plasters. It tends to affect adults who have built up an allergy to that substance after either a single or a prolonged contact with it.

Contact eczema is more complex than a straight-forward acute reaction, as the rash and itching, which appear at the exact spot where the substance touched the skin, are often delayed, but the principal mechanism involved is an acute response.

As with other allergic reactions, once a person becomes sensitized to a particular substance, memory cells are created and, whenever the skin comes into contact with it again, antibodies are released and inflammation occurs.

Occupational eczema occurs when people become sensitive to a substance they come into contact with at work. The problem may take some time to develop, often arising only after a person has been using the substance for a number of years. Essentially, though, the parts of the body which touch the offending substance are affected, most commonly the hands, from handling chemicals or wearing latex gloves, although over a long period the eczema may spread. The condition improves if the sufferer either stops using the product or goes on holiday.

Urticaria (hives, nettlerash)

Acute urticaria comes on very quickly and lasts either hours or days. Caused by a number of possible substances – for example foods, medicines, inhaled substances, or stings – there are several forms of urticaria, but the main symptom is widespread swelling and itching of the skin.

Angio-oedema, a type of urticaria that affects children more than adults, involves swelling, particularly of the face, lips, eyelids, tongue and throat, although other parts can be affected. There is a burning, rather than an itching feeling. This is most commonly due to a food allergy or intolerance and it can come on within seconds of the food entering the mouth. With treatment it settles in a few hours.

Gastrointestinal reactions

Classic food or medicine allergies may take the form of an acute reaction. Almost immediately on swallowing the substance – or sometimes just after putting it in the mouth – the allergic sufferer reacts with stomach pain, diarrhoea or violent vomiting. Skin reactions, such as urticaria, may also occur and, in very extreme cases, anaphylaxis (*see box*, page 5). In some children with a severe allergy, even just touching the item – for example, an egg – can bring on symptoms such as a rash or breathing difficulties.

Intolerances to foods are many and varied, including both the physical and emotional symptoms listed in Chapter 1 (*see page 8*). These may come on gradually, unbeknown to the sufferer and, ironically, the substance to which one is intolerant is often a favourite food, or something which is eaten very often. For example, reactions to fish are particularly high in countries where it is part of the staple diet.

Sometimes a threshold of symptoms may be reached, so that the person feels unwell almost constantly with little fluctuation in symptoms between contacts with the substance causing the reaction. This occurs when the food is eaten frequently with no time to recover between reactions. With a substance like coffee, this effect is particularly evident. A sufferer may be highly habituated to coffee, and may drink so many cups throughout the day that the symptoms simply build up to a constant level, hardly falling or rising in between cups, and making it almost impossible to find the connection between the coffee and the symptoms.

'Masking' is due to a delayed reaction, and may go on for some time so that the pattern of eating and reacting is disrupted. The sufferer gets a delayed 'hit' after eating the problem food and is just recovering as he or she eats it again, so getting the impression that the food is improving the symptoms rather than causing them. Favourite snack foods, such as chocolate, are particular culprits for this, as they are eaten or drunk so frequently that the reaction to them cannot be traced back easily.

Emotional symptoms

Some practitioners believe that intolerances can cause emotional symptoms, too. Quite apart from the stress and depression the sufferer naturally feels because of a chronic condition, practitioners say that some intolerances can cause panic attacks, depression, mood swings, aggression, irritability and other changes to the sufferer's personality. These cannot be treated effectively with conventional medicine as it does not address the root cause of the problem, but a number of complementary therapies may help (*see* Chapter 8).

CHAPTER 3

Causes and trigger factors

Every allergy or intolerance is a very individual reaction, and there are endless substances to which people can become allergic or intolerant. If your reaction is immediate, or takes place within minutes of eating a food, swallowing a pill or walking in the open air on a sunny day, you will not have much difficulty in pinpointing the cause. However, it may not be that clear-cut, or there may be more than one possible cause. Certain substances commonly cause allergies or intolerances, and it may be worth considering them among your first list of suspects, even if you later eliminate them from your inquiries.

What causes allergies and intolerances

Three main groups of substances cause allergies or intolerance. These are known as allergens:

- those that are in the air and inhaled, such as pollen or dust (aeroallergens);
- those where physical contact causes an allergic reaction – for example, nickel, latex and certain chemicals;
- those that cause a reaction when eaten, such as foods or certain drugs like penicillin or aspirin, both common allergens.

Sometimes the symptoms caused by a specific allergen

seem to have a logical connection, such as allergy to inhaled pollen causing hay fever, or a rash appearing where a piece of costume jewellery touches the skin, but it is not always that straightforward. Food allergies can cause rashes and breathing problems, for example, so the allergy sufferer, or his or her parents need to be very observant in order to detect the substance or substances which trigger the allergic reaction.

Allergies and intolerances caused by inhaled substances

Most of these are acute reactions which cause the typical symptoms outlined in Chapter 2. Hayfever or rhinitis is probably the commonest of the allergies caused by inhalation. As many atopic asthma sufferers also suffer from rhinitis, the inhaled allergens affecting both groups are largely the same.

Main causes of allergy caused by inhalation

Pollen
Grasses
Trees
Plant sap
Organic dust (from timber, flour)
Mould (spores, fungi and vegetation outside; humidifiers, mould and mildew indoors)
Cigarette smoke
Fumes (pollution or chemicals)
Animals (furry pets, especially cats, are a particular problem)
Birds
House dust mite

The main difficulty with an allergy or intolerance to inhaled substances is that it is almost impossible to avoid breathing in small particles in the air, so often it is not possible to eliminate a substance to which you are allergic or intolerant. Fortunately, many television and radio stations and newspapers now announce the local pollen count (the concentrations of pollen in the air) and the air quality for the day ahead, which at least can help asthma and hay fever sufferers to plan and, if conditions are going to be particularly uncomfortable, to take precautions or even to stay indoors.

Outdoor allergens

The term hay fever is misleading, because the condition is caused by pollen, not hay. A more accurate term would be seasonal allergic rhinitis, and some unfortunate people suffer from sniffles all year round, a condition known as perennial rhinitis. Sufferers from atopic asthma will find that they are sensitized to many of the same substances.

Grasses and other plants with fine pollen scattered by the wind are the main culprits for causing rhinitis and asthma attacks, as the pollen can travel a long distance. Allergic and intolerant people have a reaction when the concentration of pollen reaches a certain threshold, usually 10–20 grains per cubic metre of air. On 'bad' days in summer this can reach 100–500! Those plants with bright flowers and large seeds, which are carried by insects, tend to be less allergenic, although some very sensitive people may experience a reaction to them.

Other plants can cause rhinitis, too. In autumn particularly, fungi and spores are a significant problem.

Common plants causing hay fever

Gramineae (grasses)
Ragweed (the biggest offender in the USA)
Couch grass
Rye grass (in many English lawns)
Reeds
Meadow grass
Rye
Oats
Wheat
Meadow fox-tail
Trees
Birch
Maple
Alder
Hazel
Beech
Elm
Willow
Poplar

Herbaceous plants
Dandelion
Daisy
Plantain
Artemisia
Sheep-sorrel
Nettle
Goldenrod

Indoor allergens

Tucked away in our nice warm homes, we are still not free of the threat of inhaled allergens. The cosy environment of a modern house is a haven for indoor pollutants, humidity, dust and pet dander, all of which contribute to allergies and intolerances.

A damp, mouldy indoor environment can spark off an allergic reaction and humidifiers installed in some homes have also been seen to bring on attacks of asthma or rhinitis. Condensation from washing drying indoors and in kitchens and bathrooms can have the same effect.

Modern homes hide other threats, especially 'outgassing' from certain building materials, preservatives, man-made insulating and furnishing materials and fibres. Central heating boilers (particularly gas) and poorly maintained gas fires and cookers may give off nitrogen dioxide fumes which can cause asthma.

Our homes are full of internal pollutants which disperse particles into the air we breathe. These include air fresheners, aerosol propellants in deodorants and cleaning products, and home improvement products such as paints, glues, varnishes and solvents. Do-it-yourself (DIY) in itself often sparks off an allergy, since frequently it creates dust through sawing or drilling, and may involve using any of a wide variety of chemicals. Those with a strong smell, like gloss paint, are particularly likely to cause a reaction in sensitive people.

It is important to keep the house well ventilated and to allow any fumes to escape – bear in mind, though, that wide open windows let in pollen and other allergens from outside, so go easy on the fresh air if you react to these as well.

The house dust mite

Household dust is a common cause of respiratory allergy, and even the cleanest homes have some of this. Vacuuming and dusting can cause an asthma sufferer great distress and for some these chores become impossible.

However, it is the dust that you do not see as much as the dust that you can which causes the problems. The main drawback with dust is that it is the home of one of the commonest and most potent allergens, the house dust mite. It is estimated that around 80 per cent of people with any allergy, and 90 per cent of asthmatics, are affected by these minute creatures.

There are several types of house dust mite, but the two which cause us most problems are *Dermatophagoides pteronyssimus* and *Dermatophagoides farinae*. The mite is a tiny creature of the acarid family, around 0.3mm in length and invisible to the naked eye. Related to ticks and spiders, it likes to live in dust harboured within warm, humid environments such as carpets, mattresses, blankets, curtains and soft furniture. Our warm, centrally heated modern homes create a perfect environment for it. Chapter 4 discusses ways in which the mite can be combated.

Pets and other animals

It is common for atopic people to experience reactions to animals. Contrary to popular belief, it is not really the fur that causes the problems. In just the same way as with hay fever, the 'dander' – that is, microscopic particles of skin and faeces – sets off the allergic reaction with the effect that sufferers feel a tightness in the chest, have difficulty in breathing, and experience running eyes and nose and, occasionally, a rash. A sufferer may react to the animal even when it is not in the room, and may even experience reactions days and weeks after the animal has been removed. There is no totally safe pet, as even reptiles may cause sensitization in sensitive people.

Smoke

The link between smoking and lung disease is now without question, and it goes without saying that those with asthma of whatever type should not smoke.

Passive smoking, too, is a serious problem for all atopic diseases. If a mother smokes during pregnancy there is a high chance that her baby will develop an allergic tendency, and children living in homes where their parents smoke also have a higher chance of developing asthma and other lung disease. Smokers and people who inhale others' smoke at work are also likely to develop asthma and allergies to cigarette smoke. Smoke from car exhausts may bring on breathing difficulties, and heavily polluted industrial areas often lead to pockets of asthma.

Contact allergies

Contact allergies tend to be a delayed reaction, which usually appears one or two days after contact with the substance to which the sufferer is allergic. However, it may take as long as seven days to appear. A contact reaction is usually fairly easy to recognize because the rash and inflammation appear at the exact spot where the skin has been in contact with the allergen. The redness may continue for a few days, even if the offending item is removed, but disappears after that. It returns each time there is contact. Unfortunately, although it may start out only at the point of contact, over time the eczema may spread further afield and affect other parts of the body. Furthermore, once someone has developed a contact allergy to one substance, they may well begin to develop sensitivities to others. Atopic people are particularly prone to developing contact allergies, and these may be more pronounced when the sufferers are under stress.

Common contact allergens

The following common substances are classic allergens and affect a large number of people:

- Nickel: this is found in jeans buttons, costume jewellery, in some stainless steel and therefore in many household and office items
- Chrome
- Clothing: synthetic fibres, such as nylon; wool, including lanolin, made from wool fat, which is found in many creams and ointments
- Cosmetics, such as makeup, nail varnish, toothpaste, soap and bath/washing products. Hair products are a particular culprit, and allergy to the substances in shampoos, setting lotions and hairsprays have meant the end of a career for many hairdressers
- Medicines, such as topical antibiotics (which are put on the skin); local anaesthetics
- Pets and plants
- Cleaning products, polishes, detergents
- Certain woods, glues, and other chemical substances used in industry
- Newsprint
- Allergy to latex is growing more common, as mentioned in Chapter 1, and is causing problems for people such as medical professionals who wear rubber gloves for their work. It may also cause a reaction to elastic and many other household and office items containing rubber. Contraceptives have caused problems in some unfortunate cases

Food allergies and intolerances

Any food can cause an allergy or intolerance, but, as described in Chapter 2, frequently eaten foods are often the ones to which susceptible people, especially children, become sensitized. It is mainly the proteins within the foods that the body perceives as an enemy.

One of the main problems with food allergies and intolerances is that nowadays so much food is processed and packaged, with the result that a large number of ingredients are concealed within an apparently simple dish.

Common problem foods

Many of the following foods are extremely common in the Western diet and frequently may play a part in causing either an acute allergy, with immediate symptoms, or an intolerance:

- Dairy products: milk, cream, cheese, and any food made using these
- Eggs
- Fish and shellfish
- Red meat
- Chicken
- Nuts, especially peanuts; cashew nuts (there have been recent cases of death from anaphylaxis similar to those that have resulted from people eating peanuts); brazil nuts
- Grains, particularly wheat, which contains the protein gluten. Corn is a common culprit
- Citrus fruits
- Yeast
- Soya: many babies found to be allergic or intolerant of cow's milk have been transferred to soya milk, but some then react to that too
- Coffee may cause either allergic reactions or a chemical reaction to the caffeine – which is found also in chocolate, colas and tea

Additives

Perhaps almost as common as straightforward allergies and intolerances to foods is allergy to or intolerance of certain additives which are used to enhance the flavour, preserve it for longer and make it look more colourful and appetizing. Their longer-term effects are yet to be evaluated. Additives in food have been blamed for a number of adverse effects from allergy to hyperactivity in children and antisocial and criminal behaviour. The jury is still out on the latter, but there is no doubt that some additives do cause sensitivity in some individuals.

The flavour enhancer monosodium glutamate, which is found in many Chinese dishes, is a particularly common allergy source, and the yellow colouring agent tartrazine has also been proved conclusively to have a role in causing allergic reactions.

There is still a great deal of work to be done on the adverse effects of additives, particularly on children, who are the biggest eaters of processed foods.

Chemicals

There are two main classes of chemicals which we consume and which may cause allergies and intolerances: drugs and chemicals within food. Certain drugs have been particularly blamed for causing allergies. The antibiotic penicillin, widely used to treat bacterial infections, has been found to cause allergy in some people, and other related antibiotics may do so too. The painkiller aspirin, which is very widely used, may also cause allergy.

With our food we take in chemicals that are sprayed on crops or fed to animals. In today's society we are carrying an enormous chemical load. Not only are we breathing in smoke and fumes, handling and working with some very nasty chemicals on a daily basis, but we are also consuming large quantities of chemicals in our foods without really being aware of them. Pesticides and coatings sprayed on grains and fruit, and antibiotics, hormones and other drugs fed to animals all find their way into the food we eat, and may be contributing to the upsurge in the amount of allergic and intolerant conditions we are now seeing.

Finally, even our drinking water may be adding to the problems. In many parts of the world 'clean' water is in fact chock-full of chemicals used to 'purify' it. Other nasty substances are in there too: effluent from factories gets into rivers, and we frequently hear of 'leaks' from big plants contaminating large areas of lakes and rivers. Agriculture plays its part too, as nitrates from fertilizers seep down into the land to reach the water level. As a large volume of water is recycled these days in cities, it too is full of chemicals.

Reducing the chemical load that our bodies are suffering would go a long way to help not only those suffering from allergies and intolerances but also would help to reduce the large number of 'diseases of civilization', such as heart disease, cancer, and other problems that conventional medicine has difficulty in solving. We don't yet know the full effects of these substances on our bodies but we need to find out before even more lasting damage is done.

Conclusion

The substances outlined in this chapter are merely the commonest causes of allergies and intolerances; the list is growing constantly. The next chapter looks at ways in which you can reduce your exposure to them, and improve your health to make you more resistant to developing allergies and intolerances.

CHAPTER 4

How to help yourself

In allergy, perhaps more than in any other disease, there is a great deal that the sufferer can do to improve his or her condition. By altering your behaviour, work or eating habits, you really can make a huge difference to the problem. Furthermore, there is plenty you can do to improve your general health and well-being, so reducing your underlying tendency to react.

In some cases, once you have discovered the cause of your symptoms, it is a straightforward matter to avoid your particular allergen, be that a washing powder, fabric or type of food. Sometimes, however, it may not be that easy. With the best will in the world, and the most stringent cleaning programmes, it is just not possible to eliminate all particles from the air, nor may it be realistic to avoid all contact with a particular chemical or product with which you work. Nonetheless, even if you cannot avoid the cause of your allergy or intolerance completely, there is a great deal that can be done in the short term to reduce your exposure to it and, in the long run, to create and maintain an optimally healthy mind, body and spirit, with a strong immune system.

First, you should find out the cause of your problems. Doctors and other people specializing in allergy can carry out tests, but initially there are a few things you can do yourself to try to identify your own allergen.

Finding the cause of your allergy

Most people with allergies or intolerances have probably been trying for some time to identify the cause of their symptoms. Those who suffer from a straightforward acute (immediate reaction) allergy should have a good idea of this as the reaction is prompt following exposure to the allergen. This is more difficult for chronic sufferers because the reactions may be delayed or masked (*see* page 18) and may not apparently be linked with a specific event. If the allergy or intolerance makes you really unwell, you should seek professional help, but if you want to start with some self-help detective work, there are some key questions you can ask yourself.

Key questions to ask yourself about your allergy or intolerance

When do the symptoms come on?
Is there anything that improves them or makes them worse – eg, vacuuming, gardening, outdoor exercise?
How long do the symptoms last?
Are they worse at certain times of the day?
At work?
At home?
During the week or at weekends?
On holiday? If so, are they better by the sea where there is less pollen?
Does the time of year or the weather affect them?
Have you a pet? Are your problems worse when it is around?
Are there any smells you particularly dislike?
Are there any foods you particularly like, even crave, or cannot bear to do without?

The answers to these questions probably won't solve

your allergy or intolerance, particularly if you have a long-term problem, but they may give you some pointers as to where to start looking. If your symptoms are much better at the weekends and on holiday, it is a fair assumption that something at work is causing the problem. If, on the other hand, you find that you react more at home, in the summer months, and especially when you have been outdoors, you can start looking there for your allergens.

Don't forget that some signs may be misleading – foods can cause respiratory problems, for example, not just airborne allergens, and chemicals or other substances can cause gastrointestinal (stomach) reactions, so you may need to think laterally and to keep an open mind about the cause of your allergen. It is important to remember that you may get a few false starts; some clues may be misleading, but that is the nature of detective work, and at least you will find out what you are *not* allergic to or intolerant of.

Testing yourself

Once you believe that you have identified the cause of your problem, it is time to put your theory to the test. The simplest home test is known simply as the 'sniff test'. Sit down, holding whatever substance you suspect in a container or in your hand, and take a good deep sniff. Do your eyes itch or do you sneeze? Do your usual symptoms start? If not, wait a few moments and have a few more sniffs. If you then get a reaction, you can work out how to eliminate this substance from your life, or at least how to reduce your exposure to it.

If the suspected problem is the family pet, for example, another simple test is to stroke it and then rub your eyes. Those who are allergic to or intolerant of pet dander usually find they have a rapid reaction with sore, streaming eyes and a runny nose. You can have your suspicions confirmed with a professional test, such as a prick, patch or RAST test, which are discussed in Chapter 5.

Foods

Food allergies and intolerances are often difficult to pin down for the reasons outlined in previous chapters. Except for sufferers who experience an almost immediate reaction, it may be very hard to find the link between eating the food and suffering the symptoms. The only effective way to do this is to remove the offending food from the diet, and then to reintroduce it – the challenge test – to see if a reaction occurs. This is discussed in detail in Chapter 9, but you can carry out an informal test at home if you suspect a certain food. It is important to maintain a balanced diet, so strict elimination or exclusion diets, cutting out a large number of foods, should only be carried out under reputable professional supervision.

Keep a food diary throughout the period of exclusion and challenge so that you can look back at your patterns of eating and symptoms, and try to be diligent about remembering every single thing you take. Decide what you would like to avoid – you may have a hunch as to which substance or substances may be causing the problem, and on a certain date, stop eating or drinking them. Take care to ensure that you do not accidentally eat or drink any of that food which may be concealed in another dish. You need to be sure that it has completely worked its way out of the body, so avoid it for at least five to ten days. If you leave out the food for over a month, you may start to become 'tolerant' of the food and your body may initially accept it without reaction. This does not mean that your allergy or intolerance is 'cured' – if you go back to eating it regularly, the symptoms may well start up again after a while.

If you start to feel better over the exclusion period, you may be on the right lines. If initially you feel worse, you almost definitely are. Withdrawal symptoms, especially when you give up a food which you crave and to which you are allergic or intolerant, are common, and feeling terrible while excluding them is a very strong hint that you have found your problem. After a few days, the symptoms will wane and you will feel a great deal better than you did before.

Now it is time to challenge. Take a small amount – just a mouthful or two – of the food or drink. If nothing happens, try a little more about an hour later, and so on, until you try a normal helping. If you get a reaction at any stage, you have your result. It is important, however, to remember that if your symptoms are usually delayed, it may take a while for them to show up now too, so continue to test yourself for several days to make sure that you have not missed the reaction.

Reducing the risks

We can all do a great deal to influence our own environment and, as parents, to improve the environment our children live in. This is particularly important in atopic families, where a parent and one or more children suffer from a general tendency towards allergies.

Our homes are the first place to consider when we try to reduce the levels of allergens to which we are exposed. Making them comfortable and cosy has created a haven for allergens, and it may be necessary to reduce some of the comfort for the sake of our health. It is not really such a sacrifice. While almost essential guidance for atopic families, the suggestions given below are useful to anyone who wants to reduce the allergic content of his or her environment, and may prevent an allergy or intolerance occurring in the first place.

The healthy home

As mentioned earlier, the house dust mite is the prime culprit for causing allergy in the home. The mite lives in soft furnishings, carpets and curtains, and is particularly comfortable in warm, humid, centrally heated environments, with the bedroom and especially the bed, as its favourite place.

The first thing to do is to reduce the mite's habitat.

- Replace the pillows and bedding with products manufactured from man-made, low allergen fillings. Cover the bed and the pillows with dust mite avoidance covers. These provide an effective block, stopping the mite faeces from reaching the surface. Air all bedding thoroughly and change the sheets and bedding regularly. Sheets should be washed at 58°C or above to kill any mites.
- Remove carpets and curtains. Vinyl or wooden floors and blinds can be wiped down and kept clean, so that there is no hiding place or food supply for the mites.
- Start a vigorous cleaning campaign with daily vacuuming and regular washing of the curtains.
- Avoid the use of chemical cleaning sprays or air fresheners as they themselves can cause allergies in susceptible people.
- In a child's bedroom, keep soft furry toys to a minimum, giving the child wooden or plastic toys instead. Any furry toys should be washable at 58°C to kill off the mites.
- Reduce dust throughout the house by damp dusting. Soft cushions and upholstered chairs should be kept to a minimum, and shelves of ornaments, books and

knick-knacks should be kept behind glass. This makes for easier cleaning, even in a non-atopic household. Indoor plants should be wiped well or removed altogether.

- Consider fitted wardrobes and units, and think about stencils and other paint effects to brighten the walls, rather than pictures in frames that hold the dust.
- Keep the humidity down; use extractors.
- Central heating is another cause of the increase in allergy. Relocate the boiler outside and, if you can afford it, consider underfloor heating or an alternative that does not stir up the dust. Keep the house well ventilated, although be careful not to let in too many airborne allergens by leaving the windows open for too long.
- Many vacuum cleaners puff out almost as much dust as they take in. If possible, replace your old cleaner with a model that has an efficient filter system.
- If you have a pet, keep its living areas especially clean. If you have had to give away your pet, continue to clean that area thoroughly for at least six months and, if possible, have the carpet steam cleaned.
- Don't smoke in the house. Apart from all its other hazards, smoke is a major irritant to a vast number of atopic people. A few manufacturers have hit the headlines for promoting 'low-allergen' products which have not met their claims. In the UK, the Low Allergen House (*see* Appendix B) is completely kitted out with researched low-allergen products, and this information is available on the Internet. The Association of Allergen Avoidance Products and Services can direct you to companies whose products have all been through clinical testing.

Do-it-yourself (DIY)

Home improvement (do-it-yourself or DIY) is an area where inevitably you will come into contact with a wide range of powerful substances, many of which can cause allergic reactions. Most DIY causes dust to be stirred up or even created, such as when drilling or planing, and powerful, strong-smelling chemicals may be used, such as glues, varnishes, preservatives, paints and solvents.

It is a reasonable generalization to say that substances with strong smells are likely to be irritant to a susceptible person. In that case, avoid certain DIY jobs and using very powerful chemicals but, if you must, make sure that you leave the windows open until the substance has dried and the smell reduced. Wear a mask, and certainly protective gloves and long sleeves.

Water-based paints are less irritant and better for use in atopic households – once on the walls they also give off lower levels of fumes and are healthier.

Gardens

There is no need for the allergy sufferer to be banned from the garden, even if pollen and spores are the main cause of his or her problems. Plants that commonly cause allergy or intolerance are listed in Chapter 3 and should be avoided, of course, but it is perfectly possible to culti-vate a beautiful 'low-allergen garden'.

As a general rule, avoid plants with very strong scents. Plants which are pollinated by insects have larger, heavier pollen particles which are less likely to be air-borne and cause allergy. Keep the weeds down! Gardening activities need to be carried out sensibly. If possible, have paving or gravel in preference to a lawn. If that is not realistic, try to get someone else to mow it for you, or do it in the morning when the wind is low and there is less risk of pollen flying about. Cool, damp days are the best for allergic gardeners; listen to the announcements on radio and television regarding pollen counts and avoid gardening on days when it is high – even if you have a low-allergen garden your neighbours may not and you can't stop the pollen coming over the fence. Wearing dark glasses outdoors can be helpful, and if you have a skin reaction to leaves or sap, wear long sleeves and gloves.

We use many chemicals in our gardens today – pesticides, fungicides, fertilizers, and so on. Long-term exposure to these is probably not doing the gardener any good, nor in many cases are they good for the soil or the insects in the garden. It may be worth giving serious consideration to 'going organic', or at least reducing the use of chemicals in your garden, thus reducing your own chemical load as well as that on your immediate environment.

The work environment

Your working environment is, of course, a more difficult area to control than your own home.

If your allergy or intolerance is connected with a chemical, animals or substance with which you work, a more serious problem is at issue. Depending on the nature of the allergy or intolerance, you may find that protective clothing in the form of a mask or gloves may help. You may be able to use some alternative substance in your work, or you may be able to move to a different part of the company where you will not be exposed to your allergen.

Avoiding problem foods

Once you have pinpointed your food allergy or intolerance, you will notice an improvement once you start to
avoid it. Hard as that may seem, the improvement in
your well-being and health will soon make that seem
worthwhile.

Learn to be suspicious – read the packaging on food so
that you don't accidentally eat your problem substance –
and don't be afraid to ask in restaurants about what
certain dishes contain.

One food allergy or intolerance may lead to another,
so try to avoid eating any single food too often (*see*
rotation diets, page 107). You are most likely to become
allergic or intolerant to the foods that you eat most
frequently.

It has been found that some intolerances (as opposed
to allergies) do actually fade away over time. If you
avoid your problem food for a while, you may find that
you can gradually reintroduce it into your diet in small
quantities without a problem. Don't overdo it, though,
or you may well find that the intolerance gradually
builds up again and you will be back to square one.

If your allergy or intolerance is a dramatic one and
you risk an anaphylactic reaction, it may be worth
investing in a Medic-Alert or similar bracelet. In this
you can record details of your allergy and the need for
immediate hospital treatment. That way, if you accidentally eat the food to which you are allergic and start to
react violently with no one around who knows you well,
someone can find out what to do and act immediately.

Preventing allergies

In a family known to have an atopic tendency, any new
baby is particularly vulnerable to developing allergies in

early life. An elder brother or sister who is atopic is a major risk indicator of developing atopy, and premature or small babies are also at high risk. Recent research, however, has shown that if a child is not sensitized in the first six months of life, he or she may escape altogether and grow up without a predisposition to allergies.

The main aim, therefore, is to keep the baby's environment as free from allergens as possible. This means scrupulously following the suggestions for the child's room and the cleaning schedule outlined on pages 36-7.

'Breast is best' has come back into fashion, but it is largely believed that in addition to the other benefits and protection it offers, the mother's breast milk helps to protect the baby from allergy. Allergy or intolerance to cow's milk is common in small babies, and often they also become allergic to soya and other alternatives. If possible, the baby should be breast-fed and not weaned before six months. If it is not possible to breast-feed, then the baby should be fed on infant formula. Cow's milk should be avoided until the baby is around a year old.

Protecting the future

In so many ways, we are only just now beginning to realize just how important mother's diet and lifestyle can have lifelong implications for the future health of her unborn child. Allergies and intolerances are no exception. Even before conception, the mother's diet can influence the baby's tendency towards allergy or intolerance. If the pregnancy is planned, it is more essential than ever to maintain a healthy lifestyle in order to give the child its best possible start in life. Keeping up these habits after the birth, and instilling a good healthy approach in your children, is the best way to ensure that they never know the misery an allergy or intolerance can cause.

Improve your own health

Improving your own health and general well-being is central to dealing with allergies and intolerances. The symptoms are the outward sign of an underlying problem, so if you can boost your immune system, improve your general level of health and 'think positive', your body will start to heal its predisposition to allergy. Adopting a basic 'healthy lifestyle' is the first step.

- Get plenty of exercise and fresh air, especially if you work indoors in artificial light. (Seasonal Affective Disorder, suffered by some people in the winter when it is dark, does not affect us all, but we do feel better if we get some natural light and air.)
- Eat a healthy diet, and try to use fresh, organic (if possible) food. Try to vary your diet so that you don't eat the same food or food type too often.
- Nutritional supplements boost the immune system and help to protect against some of the harmful substances to which we are exposed daily. These are available from health food shops, as is advice on them. Chapter 9 looks at the use of food supplements in more detail.
- Avoid taking drugs unless it is absolutely necessary – overuse of antibiotics, in particular, damages the immune system.
- Wear natural fabrics and try not to use too many chemicals in your home.
- Cut down on alcohol, especially if you often feel that you 'need a drink' when you come home; reduce your intake of tea and coffee. Herbal infusions, such as camomile tea, are a healthier alternative.
- Don't smoke. Cigarettes contain poisonous chemicals which have an adverse effect on almost every system of the body.
- Drink filtered or bottled water.

- Breathe well and stand tall – if you slump you don't get as much air into your lungs, and your body will feel better if your posture is good. Don't overbreathe, though; this will increase anxiety. If you are a rapid, shallow breather, a physiotherapist might help to show you more effective techniques.
- Get enough sleep.
- Consider buying some relaxation tapes, or just listening to soothing music.
- Learn and practise a relaxation technique, such as self-hypnosis or meditation (*see* Chapter 8).

Think positive

One of the worst things about a long-term illness is that it can take over your life. If you can't look in the mirror without being reminded of your eczema, or eat a meal without worrying about what may be lurking in it, it is very easy to become obsessive and to think about nothing else. It can also happen that allergic or intolerant reactions become a kind of 'learned response' – people react when they expect to, and there is evidence that some people start to experience the symptoms of hay fever when even they come close to artificial flowers.

'Thinking positive' is crucial to improving the feelings of stress and depression caused by a long-term problem such as allergy or intolerance.

The following guidelines may be helpful:

- Try to avoid situations that you know will cause you stress – look at your lifestyle and see if you can eliminate some of the main causes of stress.
- Learn techniques such as assertiveness which may help you to deal with difficult situations.
- Pursue a hobby, preferably one that gets you out and about.

- Develop outside interests, and meet new people.
- Allow yourself some time off. Many anxious people are constantly 'on the move' – for example, always doing jobs around the house when they are not working, instead of allowing themselves a bit of peace and quiet. It is no crime just to take some time to allow yourself to get in touch with your own thoughts and emotions.
- Learn techniques such as positive affirmation (*see* page 98) that will help you to feel more positive about yourself.

CHAPTER 5

Conventional medical treatment

What your doctor will tell you

If merely avoiding your particular allergen is not possible, or if you are still not sure what is causing your symptoms, there are a number of effective treatments for allergy-related problems which your doctor can recommend or prescribe. There is also an increasing number of specialist allergy centres which can carry out further tests and prescribe a variety of treatments.

History taking

Initially, your doctor – or indeed any good practitioner – will compile a detailed history of your problems, asking many of the questions about your symptoms that were discussed in Chapter 4.

In many ways, the sufferer's history is the most important single factor in diagnosing allergies and intolerances. Allergy tests can sometimes give misleading results, and if these conflict with your own experience, they should be treated with some suspicion. For example, if a test suggests that you have a sensitivity to a certain substance, but you know that you have never actually suffered a reaction to it, your medical history is likely to be the more trustworthy.

Allergy testing

Once the doctor has a good picture of your symptoms, he or she may decide to carry out an allergy test, or refer you to a specialist allergy centre for this.

Skin prick testing

Skin prick testing is commonly used to identify a number of different types of allergen, including the inhaled substances like pollen. It is normally the first approach. Once the history has given clues as to some possible causes, a drop of the suspected substance or substances is placed on the skin, usually the forearm, and a tiny is prick made through the skin with a needle or lancet. If you are allergic to that substance, within a few minutes it will become itchy, and then red and swollen – a typical allergic 'weal'. Only a tiny amount of the allergen is used, and only involves substances which are commonly around us, so it is quite safe. The reaction goes down within a few hours.

Patch testing

This is normally carried out for skin allergies, such as eczema and dermatitis. A tiny quantity of the potential allergen is placed on a patch and stuck on to the skin, usually the back. Around two and four days later, the patches are checked for an allergic reaction, usually an outbreak of eczema at the spot.

Most allergy centres which carry out this type of test have a standard 'battery', or range of common allergens to which people are sensitive, such as nickel, chromate or rubber, and more specific batteries relating to occupations, such as a baker's battery, containing extracts of grains, or for other industries, including common problem substances like oil coolants.

Blood testing

A number of blood tests are used to identify allergies but one of the commonest is the RAST (radioallergosorbent) test. In this test a small sample of the patient's blood is taken and sent to a laboratory, where the amount of IgE (the antibody immunoglobulin E) is measured against a variety of specific allergens. If this is raised in the presence of a certain substance – for example, house dust mite – it suggests that an allergy is present.

ELISA food sensitivity tests are blood tests designed to detect food specific IgG (immunoglobulin G, another antibody present in some allergies) in the serum. These aim to identify not only true allergies but also sensitivities. They were developed in the United States and are widely available there, but have more recently been introduced to the UK. They are best used as a back-up to traditional tests and exclusion diets, which are probably more reliable.

Breathing tests

A specialist allergy clinic may carry out certain further tests in asthma – for example breathing tests, using a machine called a Vitalograph to measure the lungs' strength in exhaling. Lung sensitivity tests may also be carried out by asking the patient to inhale the substance to detect whether there is any irritation.

With any test, however, it is always important to remember that your history is central. It is possible to have antibodies to a substance without actually having allergic symptoms. Even if the test suggests that you are sensitive to a certain substance, it may never have caused you a problem, and you therefore need not go out of your way to avoid it.

Medical treatments

The previous chapters have illustrated that there are many causes of allergy and types of response. As a result, there is no single 'cure' for allergy, or even a single effective treatment. The treatments outlined below can alleviate the misery of the symptoms, and indeed prevent or halt life-threatening attacks of asthma or anaphylaxis, but they do not treat or 'cure' the underlying allergy or allergic tendency. Nonetheless, they are valuable in reducing the symptoms in the short term.

In the case of any allergy treatment, however, it is important to continue to try to reduce your exposure to your particular allergen. It is no good dosing yourself up with drugs while continuing to live or work in a dusty atmosphere or let your cat sleep on the bed.

Treatments

There are two main types of allergy treatment, applying to several different symptoms, into which most medicines fall:

- Preventers: taken while the sufferer feels well, to prevent an attack – for example, of hay fever or asthma.
- Relievers: taken once the symptoms have started, to reduce their effect.

Preventers

These drugs should be used regularly to prevent the symptoms occurring. In hay fever, treatment should be begun before the individual's particular season starts, as it may take some time to take effect. Sodium cromoglycate, an anti-inflammatory drug, is used for a wide range of allergy treatment. It needs to be taken regularly to prevent attacks.

In hay fever or rhinitis it works directly on the mast cells, preventing interaction with the pollen that causes the irritation. Available in inhaled form, or as eye drops, it is safe for children to use, and so tends to be widely used for the treatment of atopic asthma in the young.

Sodium cromoglycate may also be prescribed in tablet form for urticaria and has proved to be effective in preventing certain types of immediate allergy to food. Nedocromil sodium is another drug with a similar effect.

Corticosteroids, commonly (and misleadingly) known simply as steroids, should not be confused with the anabolic steroids used by some athletes and bodybuilders to improve their performance. Another preventive therapy, these are used in inhaled form for asthma and hay fever sufferers and work by reducing the inflammation, swelling and mucus in the airways which make breathing difficult. Powerful drugs, they are generally prescribed in a low dose, at least to start with. They may also be used in tablet form at higher doses for very severe asthma or eczema. There are risks attached to the use of steroids (*see below*), but this is mainly from steroid tablets taken long-term, rather than inhaled steroids. For very severe asthma attacks, a doctor or nurse may inject a steroid.

Corticosteroid creams are a mainstay of the treatment of eczema and, again, work by reducing inflammation.

They need to be applied regularly, but limited to the site of the eczema and used at the weakest dose possible.

Many parents are particularly worried about the long-term use of steroids in their children, and they are mainly reserved for the treatment of adults. They are effective drugs but are known to have side-effects, notably stunted growth and a thinning of the skin. As a result, they are usually used at the lowest possible dose and for the shortest period of time. It is important, however, not to stop steroid treatment suddenly, as this can cause a relapse and worsening of the symptoms.

Relievers

Antihistamines are valuable in the treatment of symptoms once they have started, especially in the case of hay fever, rhinitis, hives and eczema. They work by blocking the production of histamine in an allergic reaction. They are particularly valuable in treating eye and nose symptoms of hay fever and rhinitis, including sneezing and runny noses. Most are taken in tablet form, and many are available from the pharmacist without a prescription. They are useful for mild to moderate symptoms.

One of the main drawbacks of antihistamines in the past was that they made some users drowsy; modern antihistamines, however, do not have this effect. They also work quickly, within an hour or two. For best results in hay fever, preventive treatment should be started well before the symptoms occur, so that the effect is 'kicking in' by the time your particular hay fever season starts.

Antihistamine tablets can be of value in some eczema patients, too, but creams should be avoided, as they can cause further skin reactions.

Antihistamine creams are the mainstay of treatment for urticaria, however. As urticaria may often be due to a food or drug allergy or intolerance, the first aim is to find the cause and try to avoid it. Unmedicated creams and calamine can soothe the rash. Special antihistamine creams are available for bee and wasp stings too, or, if the reaction is severe, a mild corticosteroid cream (hydrocortisone) may be given. Calming, soothing lotions such as calamine or witchhazel may be recommended to take the heat out of the sting. In a very serious reaction (anaphylaxis), involving swelling, breathing difficulties and maybe unconsciousness, the patient should be taken straight to hospital for emergency treatment with adrenaline. Stings in the mouth and in very small children should also be taken seriously and seen by a doctor.

Decongestants work locally to unblock the nose and are effective in hay fever, but should only be used in the short term.

In asthma a number of other 'reliever' drugs can be used, such as bronchodilators – for example, salbutamol, terbutaline or salmeterol – which relax the airways in an attack, and anticholinergics – for example, ipratropium bromide – which have a slow onset but prolonged duration, and again relax the smooth muscle of the airways. A wide variety of inhaler devices for both preventers and relievers is available to suit any age and level of co-ordination.

In a severe asthma attack, the patient should be taken to hospital urgently. In spite of all we know about asthma today, preventable deaths from the condition have continued to rise in the developed world. Delay can often cost a life.

Skin treatments

Coal tar is an old-fashioned treatment for eczema, but it can also be used to help itching and scaling of the scalp.

It tends to be messy on the body and stains clothes, however. Coal tar bandages are available.

Wet wraps are favoured by some doctors for wide-spread eczema in infants and small children. Bandages are soaked in water, then spread with a moisturizing cream or weak corticosteroid. The effect is soothing and may help the child to sleep.

Emollients or moisturizers are a vital part of eczema care. A wide variety of these are available. They contain a mixture of oils, fats and water, and come in the form of creams, lotions, ointments and medicinal bath oils. Their purpose is to restore the oil and moisture content in the skin which is lost through eczema. You may need to try several types before you find the best one for you. You should be aware of the fact that some people may become sensitized to one of the ingredients in the emollient, so you should watch out for this and change the product if necessary.

Antibiotics and antifungals

Secondary infections are common in eczema. If patients scratch severely, the eczema may become weepy and infected. Antibiotics may be needed to clear up the infection. Thrush (candida) can also occur if the eczema is sited near to susceptible areas such as the ear or groin. An antifungal agent can be prescribed to deal with these areas.

Cyclosporin

This is a powerful immunosuppressant drug which is used in transplant patients and in psoriasis. It may be prescribed by a skin specialist in very severe cases of adult eczema when other treatments have failed. It is usually prescribed for short courses as it has some nasty side-effects, and needs to be closely monitored by a specialist doctor. Only the very worst cases of eczema would be considered for this treatment as the side-effects would normally outweigh its potential benefits.

Food allergy

The initial treatment for food allergies and intolerance is to avoid the problem food. Sodium cromoglycate as outlined above may be of help in preventing instantaneous reactions to foods, but little medical help is available for long-term problems. People suffering from severe reactions such as anaphylaxis should be hospitalized at once, or a partner or parent should carry emergency supplies of adrenaline and know how to administer them. Dietary treatments, for both food allergies and intolerances and other allergic problems, are discussed in Chapter 9.

Desensitization or injection immunotherapy

This form of treatment of allergy was developed in the early 20th century, and is widely available in the United States and Europe. Its use has been restricted in the United Kingdom in recent years because of anaphylactic reactions, and can now be carried out only in special allergy centres with the appropriate emergency facilities.

Desensitization involves injecting the allergy sufferer with tiny but increasing doses of the allergen and aims to boost the production of antibodies to block the allergic reaction. This has been a rather haphazard technique in the past and has been associated with side-effects and sometimes fatal reactions.

The best results of immunotherapy have been found in the treatment of summer hay fever which is not well controlled by conventional medicine, and for hypersensitivity to wasp and bee stings.

Enzyme potentiated desensitization

Enzyme potentiated desensitization involves mixing the relevant antigens with a naturally occurring enzyme and either injecting it or applying it to the skin. This treatment is offered by some specialist centres and has been found to re-establish tolerance in one to two years, if it is given at intervals of between one and three months.

Neutralization injections or Miller technique

This technique is offered only by certain allergy specialist centres. It, too, involves injecting the patient with a minute amount of their allergen, made up individually for them. Here, though, unlike in conventional desensitization where the dose is increased, only a very tiny amount is used, and this amount is gradually diluted again and again, until a quantity is reached which just fails to cause a reaction. Patients are taught to give their own injections; as their symptoms improve, they can take them less frequently. Neutralization can also be achieved with drops under the tongue, which is useful for those who do not like needles.

Vaccines

As allergies act upon the immune system, a vaccine (like those used to prevent tropical or childhood illnesses such as typhoid, hepatitis, measles and whooping cough) may be effective in preventing them. Research in this area is still in its infancy, but early trials have taken place for a vaccine that may prevent peanut allergy.

The vaccine acts by blocking the mechanism that triggers the immune reaction. If further trials of the vaccine prove successful, a similar principle may be developed to protect sufferers against other allergies.

The treatments discussed in this chapter help the symptoms of allergies but, if the sufferer stops taking the drugs, the problem returns. The aim of natural therapies, described in the remainder of this book, is to improve the overall health of body, mind and spirit, thus solving the underlying problem and thereby removing the symptoms of allergy.

CHAPTER 6

The natural therapies and allergy

Introducing the 'gentle alternatives'

The amazing speed of scientific and medical advances during this century have made it possible for doctors to cure and prevent many kinds of disease. As they have learned more, and drugs and medical equipment have become ever more sophisticated, both the medical profession and the general public have thrown all their faith behind the drugs and treatments of modern medicine, gradually abandoning the natural therapies practised by our forefathers, such as herbalism and the use of essential oils and massage, rejecting them as being 'without scientific basis'.

It is only in recent years that we have begun to realize, however, that conventional medicine cannot cure everything, especially those chronic, or long-term problems such as allergies, migraines, arthritis, ME and cancer, and so people are turning back in numbers towards the natural therapies, which may have an effect both in helping symptoms and in treating the mind, emotions and energies of the body. What is more, it has been found that some powerful drugs actually do us harm, and until we really know more about their effects, more and more people do not want to risk their long-term health.

Fortunately for the developed nations, countries such as China and India have kept up the practice of their traditional therapies alongside the introduction of modern medicine, and our practitioners have been able to learn from them. Many of these therapies, such as Ayurveda from India or the Chinese medical system, are very ancient and, although they do not have much 'scientific' documentation, they have stood the test of time, and are now seeing a huge growth in popularity in the industrialized world. Many Western therapies, too have been revived or refined.

The trend is growing stronger. Around 30 per cent of Americans have consulted a complementary practitioner. Similar findings have been confirmed in other developed nations, particularly among people with chronic conditions – many of which are found to have an allergic content – for which conventional medicine has no answer.

Conventional doctors are increasingly more open to the use of alternative therapies. Many family doctors are actually trained in some form of alternative therapy – commonly, homeopathy, acupuncture or hypnosis. A growing number of hospitals, too, either offer services or advise people about therapies that might help them, and where to find a practitioner.

Mind as well as body

Many complementary practitioners focus on reducing anxiety as the pathway to good health. They believe that if the body is anxious and stressed it cannot function properly and, if one area malfunctions, others are affected too. This makes the complementary approach particularly appropriate for allergy sufferers since even if their condition is not 'caused' directly by stress, it certainly causes stress and distress which make the condition worse. As discussed earlier, an allergy may often affect more than one part of the body, so the 'holistic' approach of many complementary therapies – that is, addressing the whole person, mind, body and spirit, not just the symptom – aims to solve the under-lying problem that caused the allergy in the first place.

Why go to a natural therapist?

People turn to natural medicine for different reasons. Many start to look for other solutions because they are disillusioned by years of conventional medical treatment which has not solved their problems. According to a British survey, three out of four people who visit comp-lementary practitioners go with problems that conventional medicine has failed to solve. Another survey of patients who were visiting a natural health centre found that most had a long-standing problem, on average for around nine years.

Some people try alternative therapies as a last resort before they start a conventional therapy that may involve strong drugs and unpleasant side-effects. Others simply prefer the different approach of alternative practitioners who tend to spend more time with their clients.

Nowadays, great stress is placed on looking after our own health. We are encouraged to eat healthily, exercise and check ourselves for 'lumps and bumps', and many of us read books and magazine articles about our prob-lems. As a result, we expect to be involved in a discussion if we become ill, and are not satisfied just to be given a prescription. So some people choose a natural therapist because they like to talk about what might be the best tack for them, and they like the time the therapist spends with them and the feeling that they are being considered a whole person rather than as just a bunch of symptoms.

The principles of natural medicine

While alternative medicine takes many forms, almost all therapies share some common principles:

- They work 'holistically' – this means that they treat you as a whole – mind, body and spirit, not just as a bundle of symptoms or a machine that has gone wrong. Therapists will take into account your personality, emotions and lifestyle as well as external influences such as your surroundings and social life.
- They believe good health comes from being in balance – emotionally, physically, mentally and spiritually – and that imbalance is what makes for 'dis-ease' and illness. In some therapies this balance also has to do with a 'life-force' or energy which is thought to run throughout the body and the universe. In Chinese medicine this is called chi or qi (pronounced 'chee') and takes the form of two opposing forces – yin and yang – which symbolize the opposites of life, such as feminine and masculine, gentleness and strength, intellect and passion, cold and hot, and so on. In India this force is known as prana and in Japan as ki. Natural therapists use a variety of methods, such as acupuncture needles, massage and meditation, to activate or redirect this life-force.
- They believe that the body has a natural ability to heal itself and that the function of treatment is to help our own healing powers. Many see symptoms as the result of the body's attempts to cure itself and believe that rather than trying to cure the symptoms, treatment should work on the root cause of the problem. Because of this, you might go away with a prescription that appears to have nothing to do with what you consulted the therapist for.
- What kind of person you are – your personality, emotions and circumstances – are thought to be at

least as important as the condition you have when it comes to deciding what treatment you should have. This means that two people with the same illness may get different medication.

Dowsing or radiesthesia is a method of diagnosis based on the idea that all substances, including the human body, emit recognizable radiations. A pendulum is swung over the body's energy centres (chakras) and the way it swings is claimed to indicate strengths and weaknesses in the energy system.

Therapists may use applied kinesiology, or muscle testing, to assess weakness in some area of the body. The principle is that foods or chemicals to which an individual is sensitive cause weakening of the muscles by changing the body's electrical field. A suspect substance is placed against the patient, often against the jaw (the nearest place to the mouth), while the therapist pushes against a variety of muscles to compare the levels of resistance. Testing often continues throughout treatment to see whether the muscle strength is improving.

What is it like seeing a natural therapist?

Although they all more or less share the beliefs described above, you will come across a great variety of people in natural therapy, far wider than among family practitioners. Dress may range from formal and conventional to informal, even quite wacky. Equally, the premises can be very different. While some natural therapists present a 'brass plaque' image, working in a clinic with a receptionist and an aura of brisk efficiency, others may greet and treat you in their living room, surrounded by plants and domestic clutter. Remember, though, that image is no guarantee of expertise – you are just as likely to find a good, fully qualified therapist working at home and dressed in jeans as in a formal clinic dressed in a suit (*see* page 119 for guidelines on how to check qualifications).

The principles of natural therapists do lead to differences in approach from those you may be used to with your family doctor:

- Consultations usually take longer. The initial visit rarely lasts less than an hour, although treatment visits are more usually around 30 minutes.

- You are likely to be asked a wide range of questions about yourself, your emotions, your job, family, relationships, social life, what you eat and drink, your sleeping and relaxation habits. This enables the therapist to form a proper understanding of all the elements of your life and to assess them in relation to your problem.

- Therapy is likely to involve advice about your lifestyle – diet, exercise, sleep, emotions, and so on – as well as specific medications or physical therapy.

- Therapy will not necessarily be directed only at the problem you came to discuss, but may encompass any aspects the therapist feels are out of balance.

- Many practitioners may be trained in more than one type of therapy, and may combine different approaches, 'mixing and matching' them to suit your particular condition. Chinese herbal treatments and acupuncture are often practised together, as they offer two different ways of dealing with an imbalance; a stress therapist, on the other hand, may use a combination of relaxation techniques, counselling and aromatherapy.

- Treatments may take longer to work because they are aimed at the root of the problem rather than at just offering rapid symptom relief. This means that you may need to allow more time and patience with natural therapies, and an understanding from the beginning of the way the therapy works so that you do not become disillusioned.

- You will generally be expected to be actively involved in the healing process and start to take more responsibility for your health. Many natural approaches require you to change things in your life.

- You will most likely have to pay separately for any remedies prescribed, and therapists may well sell you these from their own stocks. They may also charge you an hourly rate for their time, although many therapists offer reduced rates for people who genuinely cannot afford the full fee.

Diagnosing the problem

Natural therapists place a great deal of importance on your 'history'. They usually want to go into a lot of detail and may ask you about your diet and habits, lifestyle, family, and even events in your childhood. But you will also come across some other techniques.

Acupuncturists will take your pulse – all 12 of them. Each pulse looks after a different system, such as the waste disposal system or the reproductive system, and its beat gives the therapist information about the energy levels there. Pulses are also sometimes used to test for food allergy. A change in beat when you eat or come close to a food suggests an allergy or intolerance. Some therapists use a special machine, called a Vega, which tests for allergies, intolerances and other problems by monitoring changes at acupuncture points, although little research has been done in this area.

Healing crisis

Most practitioners who are following holistic systems will warn you that your symptoms are likely to get slightly worse before they get better, even that old symptoms may reappear. This is because many of the systems of alternative medicine work by jolting the body's own defences to start fighting again and to throw off the toxins or infections causing the illness. Often it has to do this quite violently, which can produce more symptoms. However, the crisis is usually brief, and although sometimes it may be uncomfortable, increased symptoms are considered a good sign that healing energies have started to counteract the illness.

Does it work?

Many people will relate their success with alternative therapies, although solid 'scientific' evidence is more difficult to come by. However, the body of evidence for the success of many treatments is growing year by year. Researchers at Glasgow University, Scotland, for example, have proved the effectiveness of homeopathic remedies for hay fever and asthma using the stringently controlled trials used by pharmaceutical companies. But there are key difficulties in testing alternative medicine in conventional ways.

Scientific trials usually compare a group of patients who are given one standardized treatment with a group given a placebo or 'fake' treatment. However, in alternative medicine, treatments are rarely the same for different individuals because therapists take into account all sorts of features, not just the symptoms, before they prescribe a remedy. Furthermore, many therapies, such as hypnosis, meditation and acupuncture, do not involve medication at all and so cannot be replaced by a fake.

On the other hand, it is important to remember that an allergy or intolerance is a chronic (long-term) problem which may improve at some times and be worse at others, and is influenced strongly by what else is going on in your life – your eating habits and other variables, even the weather. It may be that you start a therapy just as you change your washing powder, the weather grows cooler, or you simply happen not to eat a certain food for a few weeks. It may appear that the treatment is working marvellously but, in fact, your allergy or intolerance would have improved anyway.

Nevertheless, two-thirds of the people who were surveyed in the British Natural Health Centre said that they had experienced some improvement with natural treatments, and those who believed that the methods worked were more likely to benefit. It may be that alternative therapies are more effective with the kinds of long-term ailment often described as the 'diseases of civilization', such as stress, depression, migraine, allergies and intolerances, while orthodox medicines are better when rapid relief from acute symptoms is needed.

What do doctors think of natural medicine?

The attitude of doctors to natural medicine ranges from complete scepticism to enthusiastic use of it. While a small proportion of conventional doctors dismiss it as 'quackery' and another small (but increasing) number are training themselves in techniques such as herbalism, acupuncture, hypnosis and homeopathy, the vast majority are in the middle – broadminded about some approaches, less convinced about others, but prepared to concede that natural therapies generally do no harm and may, indeed, do some good.

The most common reservations about natural medicine are:

- The lack of conventional research into the effects of many treatments and scientific proof that they work.
- The inability to explain how therapies work in conventional scientific and medical terms.
- The possibility of missing serious disease if patients consult non-medically trained therapists rather than a doctor.
- The lack of regulation regarding qualifications and the lack of safeguards for patients in most alternative disciplines.

There are, of course, precautions to take when choosing a therapist and even after you begin the consultation. These are discussed in Chapter 10.

CHAPTER 7

Treating the body

Some natural therapies for the treatment of allergies work in a directly physical way. They deal with the problems that you are experiencing with your allergies or intolerances and aim to relieve symptoms, but, unlike conventional Western medicine, most look at more than simply the symptom which is causing you the problem. Most complementary therapies are 'holistic', dealing with the whole person, which is a particular bonus in allergy or intolerance since this problem may have many facets, with a number of possible physical symptoms as well as a strong emotional content.

Furthermore, the natural therapies tend to see the symptom exactly for what it is – the tip of the iceberg and the sign on the surface that there is an underlying problem. These therapies aim to tackle the underlying problem for, if that is solved, the symptoms will disappear. Many complementary therapies regard allergy of any kind, from food allergies and intolerances to hay fever or eczema, as an expression of a similar underlying problem or 'imbalance', so, although the symptoms may be very different, a similar general approach will be taken.

A number of therapies may be of help in treating the different types of allergies and intolerances, based on either Western or Oriental principles of traditional medicine. The principal ones are:

- Acupuncture
- Acupressure
- Shiatsu
- Chinese herbal remedies
- Herbal medicines
- Homeopathy
- Hydrotherapy
- Osteopathy
- Cranial osteopathy/craniosacral therapy
- Massage
- Reflexology
- Buteyko

Chinese medicine

The Chinese system of health and medicine is based on the principle of chi (pronounced chee) or qi, the life-force concentrated in our bodies. For the body to be healthy and in balance, the opposing forces of yin and yang must also be in balance. Yin and yang correspond to our concepts of opposites: hot and cold, male and female, dark and light, active and passive.

In health, the flow of chi energy travels freely along the 12 meridian channels that run through the body from our hands and feet towards the head. Each of these meridians relates to a different system or organ of the body. In illness or disease, the yin and yang are out of balance and the flow of energy is interrupted. Along these channels are located the acupuncture points (known as acupoints, where chi is said to be concentrated) that are used in different forms of oriental medicine and it is by stimulating these with needles or massage that the flow of energy can be restored.

Chinese diagnosis depends on a number of methods. A practitioner may take the pulses on the 12 meridians and examine the tongue. In Chinese medicine the different areas of the tongue correspond to different organs of the body, and the appearance, colour and coating of the tongue tell the practitioner about the state of that organ. Oriental practitioners also study the general appearance of the patient for signs of imbalance.

Other indicators, such as the smell of the patient's body or breath, or their preference for certain foods (which also are classified as hot or cold and may indicate an imbalance of the yin and yang forces) are also studied.

Liz, now aged 30, had suffered from severe, widespread eczema since the age of 18 months. At an early age this had been attributed to milk allergy but, although she avoided milk products, her eczema continued into adult life, flaring up occasionally, especially when she was under stress. Chocolate made her itch, too, but she still ate it occasionally.

When she was 23, the eczema suddenly erupted severely, covering Liz with a maddening, red, itchy condition which became raw. After seeing a television documentary, she decided to try Chinese medicine. The Chinese doctor studied her tongue, took her pulse and asked a lot of questions about her condition. He then prescribed for her a tea made from a selection of Chinese herbs.

'It was disgusting, especially as I don't drink hot drinks like tea or coffee – it wasn't till I went back again that the doctor said it should be drunk cold. It's not nearly so bad that way,' she said. The eczema started to improve rapidly, but Liz kept taking the treatment for six months until it was completely resolved. At first she went at weekly intervals, gradually decreasing her visits to once a month.

Suddenly, five years later, she had a new reaction – dramatic swelling and weals sprang up on her body –

urticaria. Her doctor sent her for allergy testing and chicken was identified as the cause. Unwilling to take drugs, she returned to the Chinese doctor, who prescribed a tea and a skin cream made up from Chinese herbs.

This time she also had some self-applied acupressure: four tiny herb seeds were taped to acupressure points on her ear, and she was asked to hold each in turn for a minute each day. 'You could feel a kind of pressure, and I couldn't believe it would work, but the results were very good,' said Liz. She also liked the feeling that she was involved in her own treatment.

The acupressure lasted for four weeks. The seeds were replaced at weekly intervals and the entire course of treatment took about three months. The problem appears to have cleared completely and Liz feels both healthier and more relaxed about her condition. She prefers to avoid chicken since her bad experience and does not drink milk, but she uses some milk products in cooking without any ill effect.

Acupuncture

Acupuncture, an ancient Chinese practice integral to traditional Chinese medicine, involves the use of needles made of stainless steel, silver or gold, which are inserted into the skin at the various acupuncture points, of which there are about 2,000. The needles are then moved or twirled with the aim of regulating the flow of chi along the meridian. These are of varying lengths and thicknesses depending on where they are used on the body.

Acupuncture has received considerable support from Western doctors, and many family doctors now practise a simplified form of acupuncture for certain common conditions. Traditional Chinese acupuncture is available

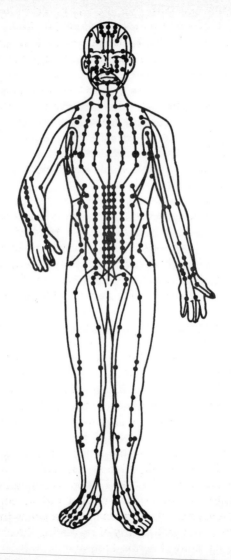

Fig. 1 The acupuncture 'energy' meridians

widely from specialist practitioners in the United States, Europe, Australasia and the United Kingdom.

Moxibustion, which is closely related to acupuncture, involves the use of the herb moxa (mugwort) which is burned close to the skin on the end of an acupuncture needle to have a warming effect at that point. Today, electroacupuncture may also be offered, which can be used for measuring energy flows at different points to locate a problem and solve it. A small electric current is passed to the patient through small metal clips attached to the needles, to find and remove blockages and to provide pain relief.

Acupuncture is a safe practice for many problems, and is said to be particularly successful in the treatment of allergies and intolerances provided that you go to a registered practitioner who follows the recommended hygiene guidance for sterilizing needles. Acupuncturists also frequently combine this treatment with other complementary Chinese therapies, such as the use of Chinese herbs.

The Chinese view of allergy, whether it is a food allergy or intolerance, hay fever, asthma or eczema, is that there is a malfunction or poor function of the liver, making it unable to process external proteins. The healthy liver should be able to moderate the outside world without overreacting to it. The symptoms of the allergy or intolerance are simply a sign that this underlying system is out of balance. Once the diagnosis has been confirmed by pulse and tongue checks, the meridians relating to the digestive system, spleen and/or the liver are likely to be worked upon to strengthen them. Acupuncture is sometimes carried out in conjunction with Chinese herbal treatments (*see below*) as these offer a different, but parallel, way of regulating the chi balance and strengthening the affected organ.

The medical profession is starting to accept acupuncture

in the treatment of asthma, although doctors insist that standard drug-based treatments should not be abandoned in favour of it.

Acupressure

Acupressure is an even older art than acupuncture, dating back to as early as 300 BC. An oriental therapy, it originated in China, but variations have been developed in other countries (see Shiatsu, page 75). The ancient Chinese found that pressure on particular points in the body could relieve pain and ailments. It is based on the same principle of meridians and acupoints as acupuncture, but involves the use of finger pressure rather than needles to restore the flow of chi to the affected organs of the body. In China, ordinary people learned the technique in order to be able to carry out acupressure at home.

Today, acupressure may be carried out with the fingers or with specially designed rollers to cover several points at once, massaging and moving generally in the direction of the meridian flow. A modern Western explanation of its effect is that the massaging action releases endorphins, the body's own pain-relieving hormones.

Acupressure is completely safe for most conditions, and is said to be particularly effective for the relief of headaches, back pain, asthma, and allergies and intolerances. It is commonly used together with other therapies, such as yoga or the use of Chinese herbs.

There are several types of acupressure, developed in the Far East, such as shen tao, do in, tsubo and shiatsu (see below), and combination therapies such as jin shen and jin shen do, developed in the United States, which use prolonged massage in combination with other therapeutic techniques.

Chinese herbs

Herbal medicine is a central constituent of traditional Chinese medicine, which has been in existence for many thousands of years. It is still widely practised in China today, both by lay people in rural communities and in hospitals, where it may be combined with other traditional therapies, such as acupuncture, or even with orthodox Western medicine.

Although they are called 'herbs', the raw materials that make up a Chinese herbal remedy may also be based on animal or mineral ingredients. Following diagnosis of the problem according to Chinese principles, the practitioner makes up a personally designed 'cocktail' of herbs to suit not only the condition but the individual patient and his or her particular yin/yang balance. The remedy is usually made up as a dried formula which is taken as an infusion, or tea, and may be adjusted frequently during the course of treatment as the patient's needs change. Depending on the condition of the patient, the herbs may sometimes be given in tablet or cream form.

As yin and yang represent opposing forces, so too are Chinese herbs classified into hot or cold, warm or cool, sweet or bitter, and prescribed to adjust energy imbalances in the patient's chi, as well as specifically appropriate to certain organs (in allergy or intolerance, the aim would often be to strengthen the liver, lungs, spleen or kidneys) and states of mind. Foods may also be recommended as part of the treatment; here, too, these are classified as hot or cold and recommended accordingly (*see above*). Although raw vegetables are an important element of many Western dietary therapies, such as naturopathy (*see* page 110), a Chinese practitioner would argue that someone with a 'cold' condition, particularly if he is living in a cold climate, should eat hot and cooked foods to restore balance. Fasting (and particularly overfasting) is not usually recommended as it is seen as risking damaging already deficient organs.

Chinese herbs may be used for young babies suffering from atopic eczema with considerable success. In this case the herbs are not given as an infusion, but made up into compresses, creams and lotions for application to the child's skin.

Shiatsu

Shiatsu is a Japanese form of finger massage, using the same meridians and pressure points as acupuncture and acupressure, but combining the technique with components of other therapies such as physiotherapy and chiropractic. The patient lies on a mat on the floor, while the Shiatsu practitioner exerts pressure on the acupoints with fingertips, thumbs, elbows, knees and sometimes feet to exert pressure. Much of the pressure is continuous and stationary. The practitioner presses and holds at the acupoints, rather than moving along the meridian flow as in acupressure, and he or she may rock the patient or move the patient's arms and legs to relax and stretch them. In Shiatsu, too, the aim is to restore the free and healthy flow of chi energy. In Western terms, blood circulation is improved and the massage helps to release toxins and tension from the organs, which is particularly useful in allergic or intolerant conditions.

As well as its therapeutic effect, Shiatsu is also deeply relaxing. It is particularly recommended for stress-related conditions, and those which are made worse by stress, which include allergies and intolerances.

Homeopathy

The principles of homeopathy have existed since the time of Hippocrates in the 5th century BC, but the therapy as we know it today was developed by the German physician Samuel Hahnemann in the early 19th century.

Dr Hahnemann discovered the principle of 'similars' – that 'like cures like' – so that a substance that causes similar symptoms to those of a disease can be used to treat it. By experimenting on himself, he discovered that taking small doses of quinine, the treatment for malaria, actually produced similar symptoms to those of malaria, so he applied the principle to other substances, such as mercury and arsenic.

Dr Hahnemann also found that the best way to avoid side-effects was to dilute the strength of the dose as far as possible, and discovered, strangely, that the weaker the dilution, the stronger its healing effect. Homeopathic remedies are therefore diluted many times over, and shaken at each stage, a process called 'potentization'.

It is still not fully understood how homeopathy works. The dilution is so weak that in some cases there are no molecules left of the original substance, and the remedy is completely harmless and without side-effects. It is thought that maybe the solution retains a kind of 'memory' of the original substance, 'potentiated' by the shaking action.

Today, there are over 3,000 homeopathic remedies available, mostly in tablet form, based on plants, metals and minerals. The practice of homeopathy is probably the complementary therapy that is most widely accepted – and practised – by the medical profession, and has the biggest body of scientific research to back it up. Dr David Reilly, a homeopath in Glasgow, Scotland, has carried out several trials along conventional medical lines which have provided strong evidence that homeopathic treatment is more effective than placebo in hay fever and asthma.

Homeopaths believe that the body can heal itself, and that symptoms such as inflammation, vomiting, runny nose, such as are seen in allergies and intolerances, are signs that the body is fighting the invading organism. As a result, they will not prescribe a remedy to suppress the symptoms, rather one that would produce similar effects in order to 'kick-start' the body's own self-healing powers. In hay fever, for example, allium cepa (based on red onions) may be used, as it causes watering of the eyes and therefore helps that particular symptom.

As homeopathy aims to treat the whole person rather than the specific illness, the homeopath will take a very full history, including various details about a person's lifestyle and mental/emotional state. As a result, the treatment of two different people with apparently the same problem may be different, and people with different illnesses may find that they are treated with the same remedy.

Some homeopaths specialize in allergy testing and treatment, offering a kind of homeopathic desensitization, known as 'isopathy'. The homeopath will test for a variety of allergies or intolerances using either skin tests or a machine such as a Vega, which measures energy levels at acupuncture points. Then, rather than treating the patient with a substance that produces a similar effect, a tailor-made remedy will be made up based on the actual substance that causes the allergy or intolerance. If desensitization can be achieved, the allergy or intolerance may be cleared in as little as six weeks.

Some standard homeopathic remedies are available in pharmacies and health food shops, including one called Mixed Pollens 30 for hay fever, but these can be somewhat hit and miss, and for the best results it is best to visit a homeopath for an accurate prescription.

Homeopathy is not recommended for the treatment of a severe, acute reaction, such as anaphylaxis, when medical attention should be sought immediately.

JOHN (HOMEOPATHIC DESENSITIZATION, PLUS DIET AND RELAXATION)

John, in his 40s, was the owner of a small engineering company. He spent a lot of time driving his car and trying to secure contracts for the business. It was a stressful job with much travelling and the need to meet short deadlines. He had been suffering from ulcerative colitis for some time, with inflammation of the intestine causing pain and diarrhoea. He had also lost a great deal of blood and had become emaciated. His illness meant that he was unable to keep up his busy schedule, thus losing him business and causing him more stress.

John was tested for allergies using a modified and simplified muscle-testing technique. Muscle weakening in the presence of cow's milk, wheat, eggs, and the car and diesel fumes from his work, showed him to be allergic to these substances. He did not react to airborne pollutants.

John was too emaciated, ill and stressed to begin desensitization immediately, so the therapists restructured his diet to eliminate the foods to which he was allergic. The bleeding stopped within a week. He was taught relaxation and counselled on changing his lifestyle to reduce his stress and strengthen his body. As his system became stronger, he began the Centre's homeopathic desensitization programme. Over a period of three months, John received a range of the Centre's own specially designed isopathic treatments, made from the specific allergens to which he was sensitized, and 'enhanced' to increase their effectiveness. He did not need to be treated for all his allergies – as the main problem areas were addressed, some of the minor problems disappeared naturally.

Meanwhile, working with him on past experiences, the therapists uncovered and addressed other sources of stress. He did not have a good relationship with his wife, who also worked in the business. John cut back on the travelling and, having moved out of the family home, found that he started to get on better at work with his wife again.

John no longer has ulcerative colitis. According to his therapists, he will probably always have a genetic predisposition to allergies but, if he keeps his stress levels under control and maintains a healthy lifestyle, there is no reason why his problems should recur.

Herbal medicines

Almost every culture in the world has a tradition of herbal medicine, practised by the people who grew and gathered the herbs. These were usually the 'medicine men' or old women, many of whom were believed to have some kind of magical power, or who even used witchcraft. With the boom in pharmaceuticals, though, the developed nations largely lost touch with their herbal heritage. Fortunately, however, the expertise in herbal medicine did not die completely and, with the discovery that drugs do not always work and may have unwanted side-effects, people are returning increasingly to herbal remedies.

Herbs that are used in medicine are not herbs as we understand them for cooking. A medicinal herb can mean any plant or flower that is used for its healing properties, many of which have been known about, even if not fully understood, for centuries.

Many modern drugs have their origins in herbs – aspirin, for example, contains salicylic acid, found also in the herb meadowsweet, and the drug digoxin, used for patients with heart conditions, is derived from digitalis, or foxglove, which herbalists used for the same purpose. A crucial difference, though, is that herbalists use the whole plant, rather than just extracting the single active agent, as they believe that its constituent parts help to balance and offset the sometimes toxic nature of some of the powerful active ingredients. The principle of 'synergism', whereby the strength of the sum of the whole plant is greater than that of the individual parts, is also important – ie, the different parts of the plant are needed to work together for the most potent effect.

Herbal remedies are normally given in the following ways:

- **Infusions**: the herbs are steeped in boiling water like a tea.
- **Decoctions**: woody parts are simmered in water, which is strained and drunk hot.
- **Tisanes**: the herbs are sold in the form of teabags, and used the same way.
- **Tinctures**: concentrated mixtures of alcoholic spirit and herbs.
- **Compresses**: a cloth soaked with an infusion and placed at the site of a wound or inflammation.
- **Poultices**: the herbs from the infusion are wrapped in cloth and placed on the wound or inflammation, and kept warm.

Although the principles of Western herbalism are quite different from those of Chinese herbalism, they are not completely at odds, and there are practitioners who are expert in both. Western herbs are often used in similar ways, for their cooling, warming, relaxing, stimulating or astringent properties.

A herbal practitioner can advise on suitable remedies for your particular allergy or intolerance, both to calm the symptoms and to reduce the stress caused by a long-term health problem. Poultices may be helpful in the treatment of eczema – for example, a poultice made with Savoy cabbage; marigold tea or ointment is beneficial for inflammation and itching; balm of Gilead helps several skin conditions; and St John's wort relieves inflammation and blistering, while deterring insects. Oregano is helpful for bites and stings, headaches and muscular pains, and for healing wounds. Camomile tea is widely available and popular for its soothing and relaxing properties.

It is important to remember, though, that herbalism is a specialized art. Some herbs, although effective when used correctly, are toxic and even poisonous if used in excess, so it is advisable to consult a practitioner before you treat yourself.

Osteopathy

Like so many complementary therapies, manipulation of the body has been practised for many hundreds of years, culminating in a modern therapy. Osteopathy is now well established and widely accepted by the medical profession, having finally achieved 'respectability' as a credible therapy in orthodox eyes. In the United States, osteopaths are also medical doctors, and are used by over 100 million people every year.

Osteopaths regard the body as a complete integrated system, with bone structure, organs, mind and emotions all closely interdependent, so that a problem in one part affects another, and throws it out of line.

Osteopathy was developed in the US in the late 19th century by Andrew Taylor Still, who saw the body as a kind of machine and believed that many illnesses are due to a misalignment of the body's structures.

Osteopathy aims to support the structure of the body so that it can work in as balanced and efficient a way as possible and use its own powers of self-healing to solve an internal problem. To diagnose a problem, an osteopath will take a patient's history and examine his or her body framework for signs of misalignment. Joints are moved and the body examined by means of palpation (touch). Muscle strength and reflexes are checked. The aim of the treatment is to encourage the body's own internal mechanisms to set in motion their own corrective function on the imbalance. Once the imbalance or dysfunction is put right, the body is in a position to start healing itself.

Cranial osteopathy and craniosacral therapy

Cranial osteopathy is a technique developed in the 1930s, involving the subtle manipulation of the skull. It is particularly effective on the soft bones of infants and children and, because it is gentle and non-invasive, is widely used in children with a wide range of problems.

American osteopath William Garner Sutherland found that the skull bones, which are separate at birth, fuse together with age, but still retain some mobility, and are sensitive to pressure. He established that if skull bones are out of their correct alignment, as may occur during birth trauma, dysfunction follows, which may take the form of immune system weakness, as seen in allergy or intolerance. Headaches, pain, and difficulties in infants such as colic, feeding problems, sleeplessness and fretfulness may also result. Sutherland developed a technique of pressing and manipulating the skull, which enabled him to adjust the flow of the cerebrospinal fluid that surrounds the brain and spinal cord – he called this 'the breath of life' – so restoring the balance and enabling the body to heal itself.

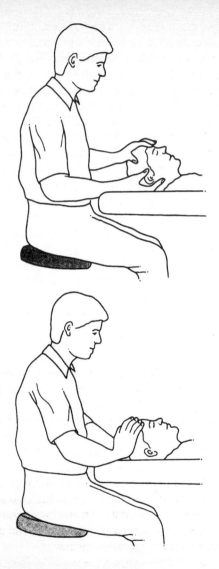

Fig. 2 Craniosacral techniques

Craniosacral therapy is a newer technique, developed out of cranial osteopathy and with similar aims, which concentrates on the flow of cerebrospinal fluid between the brain and the sacrum at the base of the spine. An even more gentle therapy, it works on both a physical and a non-verbal, emotional level, making it particularly suitable for the treatment of small children or people with painful conditions. The therapist is trained to feel for the movement of the flow and to recognize where it is restricted, which may be the cause of physical or emotional problems. By 'holding' the body at the point of the problem, the therapist enables the body to let go of its restrictive pattern, both releasing tension and freeing the energy that was previously used to contract the body.

Both cranial osteopathy and craniosacral therapy can have dramatic results, particularly in children, in whom a long-term problem can disappear almost miraculously within a single session.

Baby Lucy (craniosacral therapy)

Lucy was three weeks old when her mother first brought her to the craniosacral therapist. She was 'colicky' – uncomfortable and distressed, particularly after feeding, and generally fretful. Her skin was dry. Her mother, a strong character with firm views on parenthood, was very anxious and upset that she could not calm her baby. The history revealed that Lucy had had a difficult birth and her mother had been in labour for 36 hours.

In the first session, Lucy was tense and kept her eyes tightly shut. Holding her, the therapist was able to feel the tension from her birth trauma ebb away, and by the end of the session, she was more relaxed. The physical symptoms began to improve from then on.

At the second session, Lucy was still 'difficult' and

anxious, but her skin and colic had improved dramatically. The therapist felt, though, that the pattern of the tension had changed, and began to realize that the baby was picking up her mother's anxiety. Lucy's mother was very protective, quick to intervene if the baby cried. The area of tension in Lucy had moved and she drew back her shoulders and pelvis – a sign that she was unwilling to surrender to emotion.

In the third session, a fortnight later, the therapist tried to help the baby to release that emotion and tension, and asked her mother not to intervene. Lucy began to open her eyes and to take in her surroundings. Saying her name softly, he encouraged her to cry, keeping eye contact with her to allow her to integrate her experience.

Gradually she became more calm, and tremors, small discharges of emotion, ran through her body and her face. By the end of the session, she was more relaxed than her mother had ever seen her. The physical symptoms had now disappeared completely. The therapist explained to Lucy's mother that she need not get so concerned each time that Lucy cried or seemed unhappy – it was not a sign of her failure as a mother, simply a normal occurrence. The final session confirmed that Lucy was now emotionally recovered, and the physical symptoms, its outward sign, had been healed.

Massage

Massage is a general term for kneading and stroking the body with the hands. It provides a general feeling of relaxation and comfort, and can also help with pain relief. 'Rubbing it better' is something done by every mother, and gentle forms of massage are now widely used in hospitals and hospices on very sick people.

Depending on the vigour with which massage is carried out, it can help to stimulate circulation and the waste systems of the body to clear away toxins, and to loosen tight tissues and muscles. All these effects make it particularly effective in improving the respiratory (breathing) system and digestion – valuable benefits for allergy sufferers. Beneficial also for reducing tension and stress, massage can help to boost the immune system and will leave the patient feeling a warm glow of well-being.

Different techniques of massage have been described in several of the therapies outlined in this chapter.

Aromatherapy

Aromatherapy literally means 'smell therapy', and involves the use of essential oils. These are highly concentrated oils, made by distilling the essence of leaves, flowers or roots. Each oil has its own specific properties, either physical and/or psychological. Some are soothing or stimulant, some have pain-reducing properties and others may be used to fight or prevent infection.

Most people think of aromatherapy exclusively as a massage technique, but in fact the essential oils can be used in other ways, too – for example, you can fill a basin with hot water, add a few drops of oil and lean over it to inhale the infusion; you can put a small amount of oil in your bath or on a flannel, or use a small burner to scent the room. A wide range of oils is available in the shops for home use.

Massage using aromatherapy is growing in popularity as it is both enjoyable and therapeutic. It works on several levels: the massage action is both relaxing and invigorating and can also be used for lymphatic drainage, stimulating the body's own waste drainage system, and improving the circulation. The beneficial oils are inhaled and are thought by some to be absorbed by the skin, although the question of whether this really occurs is still hotly debated.

The aromatherapist will discuss your mood, health, diet and other concerns, and choose two or three appropriate oils. These are then blended and added to a 'carrier oil' ready for massage. This usually takes around an hour and leaves you deeply relaxed. As your priorities and situation change, the aromatherapist will make up different combinations to suit you on that particular day.

The main purpose of aromatherapy in allergic or intolerant conditions is for the reduction of stress through the massage action and the use of oils with calming properties, although certain oils are useful for both asthma and eczema. It is important to bear in mind though, that some allergic or intolerant people, especially those with skin problems, may be hypersensitive to either inhaling the oils or having them rubbed on their skin, so a skin test may be advisable beforehand. Remember also that essential oils are extremely concentrated and should not be swallowed or used neat on the skin.

Reflexology

Reflexology probably has its roots in ancient Egypt, but the therapy as we know it today is mainly based on the work of two Americans in the early years of the 20th century, Dr William Fitzgerald and Eunice Ingham. They discovered that the body is divided into certain zones and that these areas are 'reflected' (hence the word reflexology) in different parts of the feet. Pressing and massaging the relevant parts of the foot can both identify problem areas and treat them.

Reflexology recognizes ten energy lines, or zones, which run through the body and to the hands and feet.

This sounds similar to the principle behind traditional Chinese medicine, but practitioners argue that it is a different system.

In common with many other complementary therapies, reflexology takes a holistic approach, looking at the whole person, rather than just the symptoms. Reflexologists claim not to diagnose, but to locate a problem in a specific area and, rather than 'cure' it, to improve the sufferer's sense of well-being, thereby reducing the symptoms. The practitioner examines each foot in turn, applying pressure in the different areas with the hands. A sharp or tender sensation indicates crystalline deposits under the skin, reflecting a problem at the corresponding site in the body. The entire feet, not only the tender areas, are massaged, to treat the whole body.

A cleansing reaction, such as a headache or a runny nose, may take place during and after the treatment as it takes effect, but this is short-lived. For most people, the sensation of foot massage is particularly relaxing and enjoyable.

Hydrotherapy

The healing benefits of water have long been known, and the boom of spa towns across Europe in the 18th century reflects the popularity of 'taking the waters'. Literally, hydrotherapy means 'water treatment', and can be as high- or as low-tech as you like, from a hot, aromatic tub or a sauna to sophisticated mineral and massaging baths.

Today, hydrotherapy may take the form of drinking mineral waters for their health value or external treatments such as bathing, douching and taking exercise in water. Often prescribed by naturopaths as part of a complete therapy system, hydrotherapy may include the

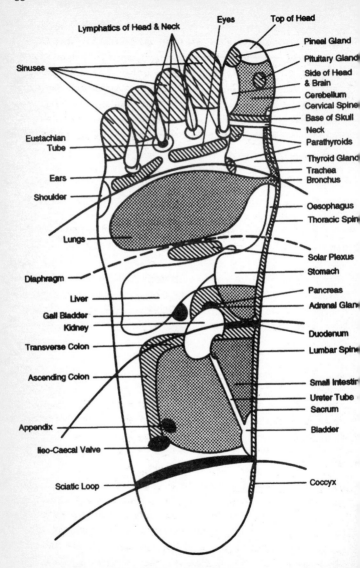

Fig. 3 Reflex zones on the right foot

use of alternate hot and cold water treatments, saunas and bathing in special baths. The alternating of hot and cold water helps to invigorate the body, improve circulation, ease pain and relax the system. It also helps to remove wastes through the skin. Some practitioners recommend the use of wet wraps containing emollients for children with eczema, which have a soothing effect on irritated, itchy skin, and can help the child to sleep. Douches and enemas are also types of hydrotherapy.

Many practitioners of different disciplines contend today that we are dehydrated – not only do we not drink enough, but what we do drink, such as coffee or alcohol, tends to be dehydrating. Rehydrating your body by increasing the quantity of mineral water that you drink may well be recommended as the first stage of many therapies.

Different types of bathing are practised today, from the bubbling, massaging jacuzzi effect of a specially designed therapeutic bath, to mineral baths, such as Dead Sea baths (particularly recommended for eczema), herbal bath preparations, and thalassotherapy – seawater bathing, including seaweed treatment. All these therapies have a physical effect, but are also soothing and relaxing. Patients with eczema should take professional advice before using certain products in their bath, in case their skin is sensitive to them.

Buteyko

Buteyko is a method of breathing which is aimed at promoting good health. Used widely among Soviet astronauts and athletes, Buteyko was discovered in the 1950s, but remained a closely guarded secret until, with *glasnost*, a practitioner left Russia for Australia, where he began to use and teach the exercises. As so few people as yet are trained to teach Buteyko, it is only slowly expanding in availability, although in the next few years it may well become more widely offered.

Professor Buteyko, a Russian physician, observed that several ill people 'over-breathe', with their breath growing heavier and deeper as they become more sick. He claimed that he could predict from their breathing when they were going to die. As a result, he developed a programme of 'optimum breathing' which, he believed, could boost the immune system and actually prevent people from developing a serious illness. The shallow breathing exercises aim to maintain the right balance of oxygen and carbon dioxide in the body. Although we inhale oxygen and exhale carbon dioxide, Buteyko practitioners believe that carbon dioxide is not merely a waste product; a lack of carbon dioxide can cause hypersensitivity.

Since its introduction in the West, Buteyko has been used primarily for the treatment of asthma, but it is claimed also to be useful for other illnesses, including allergies and intolerances, which benefit from boosting the immune system.

Breathing Control

Breathing control in general also plays an important part in the control of stress, where a common symptom is hyperventilation (overbreathing). Helping the sufferer to learn to breathe well is an important part of coping with panic or anxiety attacks.

Hyperventilation

Hyperventilation, or 'overbreathing', is due to a different mechanism from that of asthma. The person takes short, sharp shallow breaths, which reduces their oxygen level. They may feel faint and classically they experience a tingling sensation in their fingers. In severe cases, some sufferers may even pass out.

The condition is seen more in women than men, is commonest of all in teenage girls, and tends to be brought on by stress and anxiety. In people who are already asthmatic, the panic caused by recognizing an impending attack could cause them to hyperventilate, so that the two conditions coincide, or they can occur separately. The difference between the two can be detected with a peak flow meter, as the reading will be lowered in asthma but not in hyperventilation. This can be difficult to do during a hyperventilation attack, however, as the patient may be too anxious to breathe correctly into the meter.

In itself, hyperventilation is rarely dangerous as the body tends to correct itself before oxygen levels fall too low and, if the patient actually faints, their breathing will settle back naturally. The main difficulty is to per-suade some people that they are hyperventilating, as many do not recognize that their breathing pattern changes. In the first instance, it is important to calm down and try to breathe normally. However, concen-trating too hard on breathing tends to make anyone breathe abnormally, so distraction – trying to think about something else – may be a better approach.

In the longer term, learning slow, relaxed deep breathing techniques is recommended as a way of staving off attacks of hyperventilation and may gradu-ally stop them from occurring altogether.

CHAPTER 8

Treating the mind and emotions

One of the main problems with allergies and intolerances is that the symptoms may be vague and undefined, and no clear physical cause for a problem can be found. This in itself can be a very depressing problem. In addition, those who suffer from eczema, particularly on the face or hands, carry around with them a constant visible and embarrassing reminder of their problem; and the need to follow strict diets, avoiding your favourite foods, can also get you down.

A long-term problem such as allergy is worrying and, over time with little or no improvement, can build up tension in the sufferer. As a result, people who have allergies or intolerances frequently become both stressed and depressed. This has the effect of a downward spiral, as the sufferer feels depressed about his or her condition, which in turn makes the symptoms worse.

There are plenty of cases where asthma or eczema, for example, grows markedly worse when a person is anxious, either about work, school or the illness itself. When they are stressed, some people suffer allergic reactions to substances that normally cause them no problems. As the source of the worry goes away, the eczema or asthma improves. We all know that when we are mentally or emotionally 'down', we feel physically less well and, if we are happy and relaxed, we tend to feel physically better. It is not just 'in the mind' but, if the mind can be encouraged to take a more positive approach, it can have a positive effect on the body. Furthermore, some practitioners believe that panic attacks, depression, irritability and mood swings, may actually be symptoms of the allergy or intolerance itself – therapies and remedies that address these psychological and emotional problems can be of great value.

Stress

More and more today people suffer from stress. It is one of the commonest complaints that keep people off work and one of the hardest conditions to define. It may mean tension, anger, strain or excess negative energy. Some people show their stress by shouting and ranting, others bottle it up inside, getting 'uptight' with the pressure building up until it finally blows.

We all suffer from stress to some extent in pressurized jobs, traffic jams and other frustrating situations, but the important thing is to have the ability to release it. Being unable to relax, to forget the trials of the day or the inconvenience and worry of a chronic condition such as an allergy or intolerance, puts even more strain on an already compromised body, making it more vulnerable to illnesses. If you find ways to relax, or to channel that energy into positive or creative activities, the body will find it easier to heal itself.

It is important to remember, however, that not all stress is bad. Some people thrive on it and can only get things done when they are under pressure, but they have found ways to use their energy positively. The point is that you should control your stress, not let it control you.

Relaxation

For many people, relaxing is easier said than done. True therapeutic relaxation is different from going out for a drink or a game of squash – it is the complete release of mental and physical tension. There are several methods of doing this, with or without hypnosis and, ultimately, you should be able to relax by yourself, allowing your body and mind to work together at the healing process. There are many practitioners who can teach relaxation exercises, and books are available on the subject. It does take practice – you need to set aside around 20 minutes twice a day if possible, to be warm and without interruptions, so that you can practise breathing deeply and clearing your mind.

Flotation therapy

This involves immersing yourself in a flotation tank – a completely enclosed pool of salted water which supports the body, giving a sense of weightlessness. Dim light and soft music create a feeling of deep relaxation.

Autogenic training

Autogenic training is a way of programming yourself to relax at will. You learn a series of exercises aimed at controlling your own nervous system, including, for example, heaviness and warmth in arms and legs, regular heartbeat or easy breathing, so that you can carry them out whenever you want to relax.

Biofeedback

This is a way of electronically monitoring states of relaxation, such as heart rate, body temperature and brainwaves. You learn relaxation exercises and, from the biofeedback monitor, you learn how to recognize the body's own signals, such as rising stress, and find out which techniques work best to control them.

Counselling

People have always felt the need to discuss their problems – 'a problem shared is a problem halved'. In the past, with extended families, close-knit communities and a strong religious influence, it was easier to find people to talk to; nowadays, we tend to live more isolated and pressurized lives, and access to a professional counsellor to offer a listening, supportive ear is growing ever more necessary. It is now recognized that counselling can be crucial in the treatment of many chronic physical as well as obviously emotional or psychological conditions, and many orthodox doctors and nurses recommend visiting a counsellor, or even train in counselling themselves.

There are numerous approaches to counselling, but in common they offer clients the opportunity to air their feelings (often saying things they find it impossible to express to friends or family) in a supportive atmosphere. Then, together with the counsellor, they either set some goals and action plans to be implemented with the counsellor's support, or look to a longer-term aim of building up strength or health.

Psychotherapy

The aim of psychotherapy is to help people to look back at their past experiences and relationships in order to come to terms with deep-seated issues which may bring about changes in the way they think and behave. The psychotherapist, a trained listener, will question the

clients in such a way as to unravel the past and get to
the root of the problem.

Psychotherapy is particularly recommended for
people suffering from anxiety, depression or stress-
related disorders. Many people with allergies may have
had them for some time, with stressful effects on their
lives and relationships that they are unaware of. Psychotherapy can help to get to the bottom of these and, with
the help of the therapist, the client may be able to see
ways of changing his or her situation.

There are a number of mind 'techniques' that a therapist can teach to help you to 'change your mind' and to
see your situation in a more positive light. Psycho-neuro-
immunology, the medical study of how the mind and
body interconnect, suggests ever more strongly that the
use of mind techniques really can affect your health – if
you can learn to channel your mind correctly, you can
improve your condition.

Neurolinguistic programming

Neurolinguistic programming (NLP) is a relatively
modern therapy designed to help people to change their
psychological approach to certain situations. It is commonly used in business, especially in training
salespeople, and has been shown to be effective in
training people out of their phobias.

A kind of mind technique, NLP is a way of modelling
your behaviour on people who do something well, such
as selling advertising space, or coping with spiders. A
particular technique is called 'dissociation' – subjects
imagine watching themselves on a film in which they
deal successfully with their particular problem situation.
When in the future they are faced with the problem
again, they are able to trigger the memory and handle
the situation better. The technique does not work for

everyone, but for some it can have dramatic results. Some NLP is carried out under hypnosis, as some people need to 'change their minds' at a very deep level, and this can be achieved only through trance.

Some therapists claim to have had success in 'retraining the immune system' through NLP – one recounts the case of a woman who was allergic to bee stings but not wasp stings. Through NLP she learned to imagine a situation in which she was stung by a wasp and did not react allergically, and was then able to recall this when she was in fact stung by a bee. From then on, her allergic reaction was halted. (This is a potentially dangerous exercise, recounted here only as an example, since a serious allergic reaction could take place. If you have a serious or life-threatening allergy, don't risk triggering it by practising NLP at home – consult a reputable practitioner.)

Visualization

Visualization involves the use of the imagination to deal with difficult situations and increasingly is thought by some practitioners to help stimulate the individual's own self-healing abilities. They say that it has worked to halt the spread of cancers and has helped in many chronic conditions, including asthma, eczema, digestive disorders and hyperactivity, as well as psychological states such as anxiety and depression.

Subjects are asked to use their imaginations to create pleasant images, such as a rural scene (hay fever sufferers may risk triggering an attack here if their imaginations are strong enough) or a beach, in order to recall it to help deal with a stressful situation. Visualization also enables people to see themselves coping successfully in a difficult situation or overcoming their own health problems. They can look back at their past, maybe also 'rewriting' it so that traumatic events can be seen again, now with a positive outcome.

Positive affirmation

Positive affirmation involves the regular repetition of a positive message to yourself, a 'mantra', which you speak aloud. The famous mantra, that we have all heard, is 'Every day in every way, I am getting better and better,' but you can make up your own. It should be short and direct, maybe even just a single word such as 'peace', and should be repeated several times a day – for example, maybe as you wake up and before you fall asleep.

Repeating the message over and over not only encourages a positive outlook, but equally importantly the familiar repetition helps to clear your mind temporarily

---

Finding the 'secondary gain'

Without even realizing it, some people become unwell for a particular purpose – often to avoid something they do not like or because it has unpleasant associations. For example, probing by a therapist may reveal that some people who are allergic to cats may in fact dislike them strongly and in a sense have 'thought themselves' into an allergy as a way of legitimately avoiding them; or some others may have developed an intolerance to a certain food because eating it reminds them of an event or circumstance they find upsetting. Subconsciously, therefore, the allergy or intolerance offers them a 'secondary gain' – some kind of positive outcome. A therapist may be able to help to find that 'secondary gain', and look for ways in which that outcome can be achieved without the clients needing to suffer the physical symptoms.

of all the other, more negative thoughts circling in the mind.

It has been claimed that affirmation, or auto-suggestion, helps to reduce stress and depression, and may even affect skin conditions.

Hypnotherapy

Hypnosis has received a bad name owing to the performances of stage and television hypnotists causing members of their audience to perform ridiculous acts while in a trance. In fact, hypnosis has a very serious and useful function – in a trance people are very receptive to suggestion and are able to take on positive ideas, even to become insensitive to pain. Some dentists, for example, use hypnotherapy rather than injecting their patients with anaesthetics for pain relief, and other therapists use it to help people to lose weight or quit smoking.

There are different ways of inducing a trance – some practitioners may count subjects down from ten or ask them to look at a light or imagine a pleasant situation, while talking softly and monotonously. Once subjects are in a trance, the hypnotist will plant suggestions in their minds or encourage them to feel positive or self-confident. It is also a way to find the root of deep-seated problems and help the subjects come to terms with them.

You can also learn self-hypnosis techniques, either from a hypnotherapist or a book, and use them at home to stimulate a positive outlook.

Meditation

Meditation is a valuable way of enabling a person to get back in touch with him or herself. It does not necessarily need a 'religious' approach, although certainly it can be spiritual.

Meditation is an opportunity to listen to your own inner voice, allowing the mind to become completely still. People who meditate regularly can achieve a state of deep relaxation, yet with a 'passive awareness' of what is going on. Benefits can include improved concentration and emotional stability, combined with lowered stress and depression.

Flower remedies

Flowers have played a role in healing for centuries, particularly by peoples such as the native Americans and Australian aborigines, and have enjoyed a revival in recent years. The remedies are very subtle 'elixirs', distilled from the essence of the flowers, and are extremely dilute and safe. Diluted in spring water, a few drops can be taken on the tongue or in the bath. There is little scientific evidence, however, that they work.

The 'placebo effect'

The 'placebo effect' is recognized in orthodox medicine, and is a widely recorded response. Basically, it means that people feel better because they expect to. For example, in pharmaceutical drug trials, patients are asked to take either a new drug or a placebo – an imitation of the drug with no active ingredients, but which looks exactly the same – without knowing which they are taking. A small but significant proportion demonstrate the placebo effect – their symptoms improve or their pain reduces, even though they have had no treatment – they feel better simply because they believe that they have been taking the real drug.

Some orthodox practitioners claim that much of the benefit gained from complementary therapies is due to the placebo effect and that it is not a real improvement;

but the placebo effect does have its positive side, because it shows that the mind really can affect what happens to the body. Channelled correctly, it means that if the mind approaches a therapy in the belief that it will help, there is more chance that it will succeed. Whatever the reason for the success, this must be a good thing.

Flower remedies are not designed to treat specific physical symptoms but rather the states of mind that correspond to different levels of health and illness, such as fear, panic, worry, shock or mood swings. They are claimed to be of value particularly in helping people to feel calm at times of stress, and so can play a part in helping allergy sufferers who may be emotionally distressed as a result of their condition.

Alexander technique

The Alexander technique is a posture retraining rather than a therapy, but many people with chronic physical and emotional problems find that they feel healthier and more positive when they have learned and practised the technique. Most people become sloppy in the way that they stand and sit, hunching over their desks, generally slouching and slumping in front of the television. Alexander technique teachers aim to correct these bad habits. They assess a person's posture and the way that he moves, then use gentle manipulation to help him to improve the posture by altering the way that he stands, walks, lifts or sits. Twice-weekly sessions are recommended while the pupil learns the techniques. It is gentle and completely safe, and has been shown to improve respiratory function, which is very useful for patients with asthma.

Yoga

Yoga is widely used as a means of keeping fit and supple, but it has an ancient history of use in meditation and healing. Originating from India, it has been practised for over 5,000 years, with the aim of achieving physical and spiritual integration, so improving overall health and well-being. Several types of yoga exist and these have been adapted for Western use. It does not require a high level of fitness.

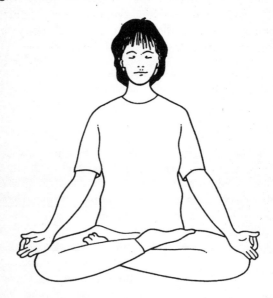

Fig. 4 The Lotus position

Yoga has therapeutic benefits for a huge range of both physical and psychological complaints, and works on several levels. The toning of muscles helps the body to return to its natural and correct alignment, which is useful for painful joint problems such as back and neck pain, arthritis and rheumatism. The deep state of relaxation that can be achieved with yoga is ideal for relieving stress, insomnia and anxiety in allergic or intolerant patients. As energy is allowed to circulate freely around the body, digestive disorders such as irritable bowel syndrome can be improved by being 'flushed through'. The controlled method of breathing to harness the life energy (pranyama) has also been seen to have excellent effects on patients with asthma and other breathing disorders.

In yoga, movements and postures are performed slowly and deliberately, together with controlled breathing, the practitioner's mind and body being focused in a concentrated or meditative manner.

CHAPTER 9

Diet and nutritional therapy

'You are what you eat'

It is widely agreed that we truly 'are what we eat'. It follows then that our diet has a direct bearing, not only on whether or not we have food allergies or intolerances but on our entire state of health, particularly on our immune system and its ability to fight infection without overreacting to other substances. Our modern eating habits, including exotic, foreign fruit and vegetables, and dishes that contain additives and chemicals, are thought to be the cause of a large number of allergy-related problems, and evidence is growing that food sensitivities may be to blame not only for certain physical ailments but also for psychological problems, including hyperactivity in children and antisocial, even criminal behaviour in adults.

There are many practitioners, both conventional and complementary, who believe that following certain dietary principles, combined with reducing our exposure to chemicals and other irritants, will boost the immune system and improve health.

Common to a number of approaches are two important principles: that we should eat 'indigenously' – that is, foods grown in our own part of the world – and in season. For example, some practitioners believe that people who live in colder climates are not designed to eat tomatoes in winter, flown in from the other side of the world. They say that it is far better for our digestion to eat locally grown winter vegetables, such as roots and seeds. In summer we should switch to salad vegetables and other crops in season.

Chapter 4 outlined the first steps that you can take in trying to identify your own food allergies or intolerances, but there are many specialists in both conventional and complementary medicine who are involved with food allergies and intolerances, and the role of diet in strengthening the body to prevent allergies or intolerances, to whom you could go.

What the therapist will do

As with any other allergy, the therapist will take down a detailed history of your problem, as well as information on your lifestyle and general state of health. Some may suggest fasting for a few days, drinking only mineral water, to 'flush' out the system. Some people with severe food allergies or intolerances may go through a very unpleasant 'withdrawal' process at this stage and, if so, it is quite likely that something in their regular diet is at the root of their problem. Often the withdrawal symptoms may be a particularly severe bout of symptoms – for example, migraine; others include aches and pains, cramps, nausea, shivers, sweating or rashes.

Following this process, the therapist will probably be able to make some suggestions about your particular possible problem foods, and will suggest that you follow a certain regime. There are many different types of diet, and the choice of this will depend on your own practitioner's approach, and the clues that she will have picked up from the information you have given. Don't be disappointed: the first foods to be dropped will probably be your favourite coffee or chocolate – as described earlier in the book, the foods you love best and eat most may well be the ones that are doing you harm (*see* Chapter 2).

Elimination diets

These are designed to identify foods to which you are either allergic or intolerant, and are a more sophisticated version of what you may have tried at home for yourself. Here again, the aim is to remove suspect foods from the diet and gradually to reintroduce them (the challenge test) to find out if there is a reaction. Very strict elimination or exclusion diets should be carried out only under the supervision of a doctor or nutritional therapist, to ensure that you are not missing out on important nutrients. There are a number of different principles relating to elimination diets, and the choice of these will depend on your therapist's preference. Here again, you will be required to keep a diary to cross-check any reactions you may have had.

The elimination diet will probably consist of a limited list of very bland, apparently 'safe' foods, to which possibly risky foods are added one at a time. A classic version is known as the 'lamb and pears' diet, so named because these are the main ingredients. The 'Stone Age diet' excludes all foods that have been introduced since the Stone Age, when man settled and started farming. It sounds restrictive but in fact allows you to eat fresh meat (except chicken) and fish, and all vegetables. The diet eliminates the eating of grains, dairy products, citrus fruits, sugars and all additives. Spring water is used for drinking and cooking, as tap water contains various chemicals and additives, and aluminium cookware is avoided. The Stone Age diet is a nutritious regime which is usually followed for around ten days to 'clear the system' before you start to test foods for an allergic reaction.

The challenge

Once the body has been cleansed, and several days have elapsed to allow all the previously eaten foods through the system, your therapist will suggest that you reintroduce certain potentially problematic foods into your diet. The return of your previous symptoms will indicate that your trigger food has been found. If the symptoms do not return, your therapist will advise you to reintroduce further foods into your diet, and what to do if you do experience a reaction.

Rotation diets

The principle of the rotation diet is that foods are not repeated too frequently, because people often become sensitized to foods they eat regularly. Rotation diets can be used both for the diagnosis of allergies and intolerances and for their treatment. Tolerated foods are eaten at regularly spaced intervals, usually four to seven days, and are not repeated in between. This does not only apply to individual foods, but to food families, because related foods, such as grains or dairy products, may cause similar reactions. A really stringent rotation diet should only be undertaken under medical supervision, but the general principle that no food should be eaten too frequently is a good idea to prevent further allergies or intolerances from developing.

Food combining – the Hay system

This is a system of 'compatible eating', devised by an American doctor, William Hay, in the early years of the

20th century. Dr Hay described allergy as 'a specific lack of body resistance to certain irritants, whether of food, pollens, foreign proteins or whatever', but stressed that 'the cause lies in the individual and not in the environment'.

The aim of the Hay system is that foods from different groups should not be mixed, and that processed or refined foods should be avoided. The result is said to be an alteration in the body's chemical balance, and the separation of different types of food prevents the allergy-causing potential of incompletely digested proteins.

The three main food groups are classified as:

- Alkaline-forming foods – for example, fruits;
- Concentrated proteins – that is, animal proteins found in fish, meat and poultry;
- Concentrated carbohydrates – that is, starches found in grains, bread and cereals, potatoes and sugars.

Proteins and carbohydrates should not be eaten within the same meal, but alkaline-forming foods may be eaten with either proteins or carbohydrates. According to the Hay system, a balanced diet consists of 20 per cent acid-forming (proteins or carbohydrates) to 80 per cent alkaline-forming foods.

Vitamins and minerals

Some people with a tendency to allergies or intolerances may have a deficiency (lack) of certain vitamins and minerals and, if these are boosted, their symptoms may be improved and the tendency towards future attacks reduced. This can be done by eating more of the foods which contain these vitamins and trace elements, or by supplementing the diet with tablets. Because of the way we grow, harvest, store and cook our foods, much of their essential 'goodness' is lost, so supplements may well be needed.

Magnesium has been found to be lacking in some people who are suffering from allergies. Increasing the intake of this is claimed to improve nerve and muscle form, so can be very useful in strengthening muscles in the airways in asthma. Zinc supplementation is particularly useful in eczema. As it is also involved in the conversion of essential fatty acids (discussed in evening primrose oil, *below*), replenishing it helps the body to carry out this process more effectively. Antioxidants, such as vitamins A, C and E, and beta carotene, and the minerals selenium and zinc, have the effect of improving many symptoms, detoxifying the body and boosting the immune system. Vitamin C deficiency is common, and boosting this is valuable in all types of allergic disease.

Bioflavonoids, such as quercetin, which is found in many green vegetables, enhance the effect of vitamin C, and help to control the inflammatory processes that take place in many allergic reactions.

The B vitamins, especially vitamin B_6 and B_{12}, are believed to help relieve asthma and food allergies and intolerances.

Consultation with a nutritional specialist will help you to decide which foods and supplements will help your condition. Some prescribe extremely high doses of vitamins and minerals as they believe that these will have a faster effect.

Evening primrose oil

Evening primrose oil has attracted wide publicity in recent years owing to its positive effect in a number of conditions, including eczema.

Evening primrose oil contains the essential fatty acid known as gammalinolenic acid (GLA). Although GLA is essential, the body cannot produce it for itself, so it is absorbed through food, for example from dairy products and nut oils. People suffering from eczema seem to be poor at converting their food into GLA, so taking it in the form of evening primrose oil bypasses that difficult conversion process. Trials have shown that it reduces itchiness and dryness, and lessens the need for steroids and other treatments.

Evening primrose oil does not work for everyone, however, and you should remember that it needs to be taken for several months and at quite a high dose (according to the instructions, which may mean several capsules a day) before it works. There has been an explosion in the market for evening primrose oil and a number of cheap, untrialled products are available. It is worth spending a bit more on a good product from a respected manufacturer as you may otherwise be wasting your time and money.

Naturopathy

Also known as 'natural medicine', naturopathy is a formalized speciality which encompasses a number of other therapies, such as hydrotherapy, osteopathy, acupuncture, herbalism or homeopathy. Practised by qualified Doctors of Naturopathy (ND) in the United States, it addresses not only the body but also the mind and emotions. The main principle of naturopathy is that the body has the power to heal itself, so treatment should be aimed at supporting the body by identifying the underlying cause of the symptoms and helping the body to rid itself of toxins. In order to do this the body needs:

• Clean air
• Clean water
• Clean food from good earth

- Exercise and 'right living'.

Naturopaths see any illness or allergy as a healthy sign that the body is dealing with the toxins and trying to eliminate them. As a result, they are against the suppression of symptoms – for example, the use of antihistamines to combat hay fever – as sneezing and a runny nose are the means by which the body expels the problem substance.

Naturopaths recommend their patients to avoid dietary stimulants, to reduce their intake of processed and refined foods, to increase the intake of raw fruit and vegetables, and to take regular relaxation. Diets such as those mentioned above, particularly the Hay diet, may be recommended, as well as some fasting. This is not starvation, just the avoidance of solid foods. Naturopaths see fasting as a way of cleansing the system and giving the digestive system a rest.

Vegetables should be organic if possible, and they should be lightly cooked in the minimum of water, as overcooking removes the nutrients. Raw vegetables and fruit are preferable where possible. Supplementation of the diet with vitamins and minerals is also recommended.

Naturopathy involves several approaches at once, so in addition to dietary change, the naturopath may concentrate on breathing and relaxation exercises, the use of air purifiers, and possibly acupuncture (*see* page 70), or hydrotherapy – the use of water for healing. This may be either by drinking natural spring waters or by bathing, douching or taking exercise in water.

Nutritional medicine

Nutritional therapy is based on the premise that many chronic, long-term illnesses, including allergies and intolerances, are caused or promoted by three main factors:

- Food or environmental allergy or intolerance
- A shortage of the raw materials which the body needs to support many vital functions. This could be caused by poor diet, poor digestive function, poor absorption – for example, because of gut inflammation – or poor assimilation of nutrients
- The presence of excessive levels of substances in the body which hinder vital metabolic functions. These might be food or environmental factors which produce negative reactions in some people – for example, house dust mite or pollen; or toxic substances, such as lead, mercury, cadmium, medications and pollutants.

Nutritional therapists aim to identify whether any of these factors are present by analysing the symptoms and carrying out skin or blood tests, and by diagnostic diets, such as the elimination diets outlined above. Having established the cause of the problem, the nutritional therapist may recommend a short period of fasting, maybe drinking only fruit and vegetable juices or eating certain fruits. This is to rid the body of the toxins and to allow the digestive system to rest. A specialized diet will then be suggested, such as a hypoallergenic, rotation or alkalinizing regime. This diet may be vegetarian (no meat, fish or poultry, but including eggs and dairy products) or vegan (no animal products at all), or one of the systems outlined above. Herbal products and dietary supplements may be prescribed. Nutritional therapists often also use extra powerful dietary supplements.

Clinical ecology

Clinical ecology is also known as environmental medicine, and works on the principle that the environment affects people's health, and that environmental stresses, such as pollution, chemicals, pesticides, and so on, weaken their immune systems, leaving them more prone to allergies, sensitivities and other illnesses. The clinical ecologists estimate that between 10 and 30 per cent of people suffer from some kind of environmentally induced illness.

As well as recommending that allergy sufferers reduce as far as possible their exposure to pollutants and chemicals, clinical ecologists concentrate on foods, the source of many chemicals in the form of pesticides, fertilizers, antibiotics (in animals), processing and preserving procedures and cooking, particularly in chlorinated tap water or in aluminium pans. As a huge amount of the modern diet is affected by one or more of these, avoiding them all would lead to serious nutritional deficiencies.

Certain dietary recommendations would be made, as outlined above, and the ecologist may recommend desensitization of the sufferer. This could mean a homeopathic desensitization (*see* page 77) or enzyme potentiated desensitization (*see* page 55).

Detoxification

It is estimated by some American researchers that as many as 25 per cent of the US population have some degree of heavy metal poisoning. Good health depends on the body's ability to detoxify itself, and people with allergic tendencies have been found to have higher than usual levels of certain metals, especially lead and cadmium, which suggests that their bodies are not able to get rid of them effectively. A detoxification programme, offered by a specialist allergy centre, might be suggested efore a specific diet is started. This might include brief periods of fasting (this is not starvation, *see* Naturopathy, above), drinking only mineral water, and the use of supplementation, particularly vitamin C, which boosts the liver and helps it in its job of eliminating toxins from the blood.

Biochemic tissue salts

Biochemic tissue salts, such as certain compounds of potassium, calcium, iron or sodium, play a part in maintaining the body's mineral balance. Made up like homeopathic remedies, in a very dilute form, the salts are non-toxic and safe to use, except by those with lactose intolerance, as they contain lactose. They are taken as small tablets. Sometimes recommended by natural therapists as part of a nutritional programme, the mineral salts can be bought from health food shops enabling people to treat themselves.

CHAPTER 10

How to find and choose a practitioner

Tips and guidelines for seeking out reliable help

Although natural forms of medicine have enjoyed a boom in popularity in most Western countries over recent years, it is still not always easy to find the right therapist for you. Once you have decided which therapy to try, there is no process like the conventional medical routine of referrals to point you in the right direction. This means that you will need to take much more responsibility yourself, both for tracking down a suitable therapist and for checking that they are experienced and good at what they do.

Finding a good practitioner, whatever the discipline, is often a matter of asking around. A personal recommendation from someone you know is a good place to start and it is even better if they can report success with the same condition as yours. If you belong to a patient support group, such as the National Asthma Campaign or National Eczema Society, you will almost certainly find other members who have tried natural techniques. Allergy and intolerance are currently very 'fashionable', and many magazines carry articles about the latest treatments. A word of warning, though – just because a certain therapy cleared your friend's hay fever or eczema, it doesn't mean to say that it will definitely clear yours. As you will know from this book, individualism is important in natural medicine and a lack of success does not necessarily mean that either the therapy or the therapist is no good. Because there are almost as many different allergies and intolerances as there are sufferers, it is a particularly difficult problem both to diagnose and to solve. You may find that you need to try more than one approach before you find the one that works for you.

If you don't know anyone with a personal experience of a practitioner, then ask your relatives, friends, neighbours and workmates. If you still draw a blank, try your family doctor's clinic. Not all doctors, or their staff, will respond helpfully and if all you get is dire warnings, ignore them. Increasingly, however, medical practitioners are broadminded about such requests. Many may have their own interests in particular areas of natural medicine and may even be trained therapists themselves. In Britain, for example, nearly 40 per cent of doctors have some training in unconventional approaches to health, such as homeopathy and acupuncture. Some clinics now have natural therapists working on their premises and in some countries certain consultations are paid for by the state health service.

Even clinics that are unfamiliar with alternative medicine may be aware of natural therapists practising in the area – if only because patients will have told them about successful treatments – and they may be prepared to give you the names of the most popular ones, even if they won't recommend a specific one. Larger towns often have a natural health centre staffed by practitioners from a variety of disciplines. As therapists usually know one another, if the type of therapy you want is not on offer, the centre may be able to point you in the right direction. Other local sources include libraries and health food shops – the names of successful therapists are usually well known. Again, if you get a recommendation for another type of therapy, try asking that therapist if they know of someone practising the therapy you want.

National organizations representing particular natural medicine disciplines, or 'umbrella' organizations that represent a range of therapies, may be able to supply you with a list of registered and approved practitioners as well as general information about the discipline. National or local associations involved in allergies, asthma, eczema, and so on, may also be able to advise you. Some of these organizations are listed in Appendix B.

Selecting a therapist

If you are lucky, you will find a therapist you feel comfortable with through direct personal recommendation. But if this doesn't happen and you have to do more research, there are certain things you need to bear in mind as you sift through the possibilities.

While most therapists are well-trained, caring and competent people, it is not difficult for crooks and charlatans with little or no training to set themselves up in practice, particularly in Britain which has almost no restrictions on who may practise when it comes to natural therapies. As a result, a British Medical Association report on natural medicine published in 1993 recommended that anyone considering attending a non-conventional therapist should ask the following questions:

• What are the therapist's training and qualifications?
• How long have they been in practice?
• Do they belong to a recognized professional body which is governed by a code of conduct?

• Do they have professional indemnity insurance?

Don't be afraid to ask such questions when booking an appointment. Anyone worth seeing will expect your questions and you should steer clear of anyone who sounds vague or shifty about answering. It also pays to be wary of being treated by someone who has done only a weekend course in the therapy they are offering.

Checking professional organizations

If a therapist belongs to a professional organization, it is a good idea to get more information about the organization itself. Some groups genuinely keep a check on their members, while others seem to be interested only in collecting membership fees and manufacturing a credibility. Questions to ask the therapist include:

• When was the organization founded? If it is new, don't reject it out of hand – ask why it was formed.
• How many members does it have?
• Does it have members nationwide? Groups which have existed for 50 years and have plenty of members may be better organized and supportive than those that started last week in someone's living-room. On the other hand, the new groups may be innovative, know all the up-to-date research and be most enthusiastic.
• Is it part of a larger network of professional organizations? Bodies representing the major therapies often belong to an umbrella organization which promotes the aims and standards of natural medicine in general. Groups that 'do their own thing' entirely may be less likely to adhere to recognized professional and ethical standards.
• Does it accept only members with recognized qualifications? If so, what are those qualifications? (*See below*

for questions to ask.) Large professional bodies may be linked with colleges which train therapists or set standards to oversee training. However, beware of organizations whose executives are closely allied with one particular school or college – their assessment of qualifications may not be independent.

- Does it have a code of ethics, a schedule of standards, a complaints mechanism and disciplinary procedures for members who fail in the standards?
- Is it a charity, educational trust or private company? Charities should promote the therapy and service interests of the public in a non-profitmaking way. Private companies are generally more interested in financial rewards.
- Are members covered by a professional indemnity insurance against accident and malpractice? This is an important safeguard and points to an overall pro-fessionalism and concern for patient welfare.

Checking training and qualifications

You may want more details about therapists qualifi-cations; in which case, further questions are necessary. Do the letters after their names just mean that they belong to an organization or do they indicate in-depth study? Information from the therapists' organization may explain this and what the recognized qualification is, or the therapists may have a patient's information leaflet. If neither of these is available, you need to ask the following questions:

- How long is the training?
- Is it full- or part-time? If it is part-time, is the training time in the end equal to a full-time course or is it a short cut ?
- Does it include seeing patients under supervision?

Qualifications which are purely theoretical do not tell you much about someone's ability to treat people and make it less likely that the therapist has had a substantial training.

- Is the qualification recognized? If so, by whom? The really important thing to know is whether the qualifications are recognized by an independent authority, not just the school or college which supplies the training.

Making the choice

Once you have found out all you can about the therapist's background, making the final choice really comes down to intuition and trying him out. The luxuriousness of the premises may suggest that someone is popular and financially successful, but it doesn't necessarily tell you that he is good. But if the surroundings feel 'wrong' or the therapist or practice staff make you feel uncomfortable, then be guided by your feelings – don't be afraid to cancel appointments, or even leave, if you don't feel happy with the person, the place or the treatment.

Precautions

If you need to undress for the therapy, feel free to ask for someone of the same sex to be present if this makes you feel more comfortable. If the therapist says no, you should leave. It goes without saying that any sexual advances made by a therapist are unethical, but if anything makes you uneasy on that score, leave at once. If a therapist wishes to touch you on your breasts or genitals, she must seek your permission first.

Don't stop any conventional drug treatments suddenly without first discussing it with your family doctor. Be wary if you are not asked what medications you are taking, and be especially wary of a therapist who tells you to stop taking any medication that has been prescribed by your doctor. Certain medicines – for example, steroids in the treatment of asthma – could be life-saving, and certainly should not be stopped suddenly. Responsible therapists and family doctors should be happy to discuss you and your medication with each other.

The medical profession has criticized particularly certain therapists' recommendation of very restrictive exclusion diets, which in some cases have led to the patient becoming deficient in important nutrients. Beware if your practitioner suggests a huge range of possible suspect foods and asks you to avoid them all at once. This is probably not necessary and may even be dangerous. If your experience tells you that you have never had a problem with those foods, then you should not give them up all at once. Sometimes a blood test may suggest that you have antibodies to a certain substance that you were unaware of. Here, too, if those antibodies have never caused an allergic reaction, you need not go to great lengths to avoid the substance.

Query any suggestion that you should pay for allergy tests and treatment in advance. Obviously, with busy clinics you may need to book sessions in advance, and a therapist may suggest that a certain number of sessions will be needed, but you should be able to cancel, without penalty, sessions that prove unnecessary so long as you give adequate notice. Occasionally a therapist may ask for advance payment for special tests or medicines, but check carefully exactly what it is for and obtain a detailed receipt.

Beware of anyone who 'guarantees' you a cure. There is no such thing.

What to do if things go wrong

The most common reason why people feel dissatisfied
with a therapist is that the treatment has not made them
better. If this happens, the first thing to ask yourself is
whether you gave it a fair trial. Did you go into it with
a positive outlook? Did you follow all the recommendations? Did you keep going for long enough? Many
natural therapies need time to work and some may even
make you feel worse before you get better.

Next, do you feel that the therapist was genuinely
trying to help? No therapy – conventional or unconventional – can guarantee success. Remember, too, that
allergy or intolerance is a complex individual condition
and therapies work at an individual level, so the one that
works for your friend may not work for you. However, if
you feel that the therapist was incompetent, caused you
harm, took risks or acted unprofessionally or unethically
– whether the treatment has been successful or not – you
should do something about it, if for no other reason than
to protect future patients.

Discuss your concerns with the therapist if you feel
you can – she may be unaware of the problem and only
too ready to put it right once it is pointed out. If the
therapist works in a centre or clinic, you may feel that it
is better to tell the management who have a duty to treat
complaints seriously and discreetly. If this doesn't solve
the problem, report the practitioner to her professional
body. This is where choosing a practitioner who is a
member of a body with a code of conduct can prove
important, although in Britain the majority of such
bodies have little regulatory power and cannot stop
someone practising, although they may expel the practitioner from the organization.

Voice your concerns to whoever recommended the
therapist to you, and to anyone else who may be affected

by his practice. Ultimately, bad publicity can be the most effective sanction, but be careful here: think through your complaint carefully and try other approaches first – making allegations without good reason may land you in court.

If you believe that you are entitled to compensation, you will need the help of a lawyer, consumers' or citizens' rights association for advice on suing the therapist – be prepared for this to be expensive. If a criminal action is involved, go to the police first.

Conclusion

Despite the occasional tabloid headline, most natural therapists are caring, reputable professionals who have invested much time and money in their training and who put great effort into their practice. Many spend just as long training as conventional doctors and are equally dedicated, although often they are not so well paid.

There is an onus on you as the patient to choose carefully and to find out as much about the therapy as you can beforehand. But this is no bad thing. Taking responsibility for your own health, searching out the right therapist and being actively involved in treatment can be an important part of the healing process. Of course, it is also in the end up to you to decide whether the treatment is helping and whether to continue. But if it isn't, do not give up hope – a different approach may work wonders. In allergy or intolerance there is no categorical right answer which is the same for every person. It is important to choose a therapy – and a practitioner – that suits you and your lifestyle and, even if your allergy or intolerance problem cannot be solved quickly, a wide range of options is available to reduce the symptoms, boost your immune system and help you to feel healthier and more relaxed.

Glossary of words connected with allergy or intolerance

Acute
Immediate, short-term and severe – for example, a reaction that occurs straight after exposure

Allergen
Substance that causes an allergic reaction

Allergy
An excessive response by the immune system to a substance which is not normally harmful

Anaphylaxis
Extreme allergic reaction involving the whole body and which can be life-threatening

Antigen
An external substance which invades the body and provokes a reaction in the immune system

Antihistamine
A drug which suppresses the production of histamine, produced in an allergic reaction

Atopy/atopic
A hereditary predisposition to allergy

Challenge
To reintroduce a suspect food into the diet after a period of avoidance, to test if it causes a reaction

Chronic
Long-term – for example, a lasting problem provoked by an allergy

Corticosteroids
anti-inflammatory drugs used in

severe allergies – for example, asthma or eczema to prevent attacks

Histamine	Chemical released by the mast cells in an allergic reaction, causing swelling and itching
Holistic	Dealing with the 'whole person' – that is, mind, body and spirit
Hypersensitive	Allergic
Immune system	The body's defence mechanism against disease and infection
Immunoglobulin	A group of proteins formed in response to invading external substances
Immunotherapy/ Desensitization	Treatment by vaccination of increasing doses of an allergen to reduce the body's 'sensitivity' or allergy to it
Mast cell	Cell which becomes activated in an allergic reaction, releasing chemicals which cause symptoms (*see* histamine, *above*)
Neutralization	Treatment by vaccination of decreasing dilutions of an allergen to reduce sensitivity
Rhinitis	Inflammation of the nose, throat and eyes in response to an allergen; hay fever is seasonal allergic rhinitis
Sensitization	First exposure to an allergen, which 'primes' the immune system to mount an immune response when the allergen is encountered again
Topical	At the site of the problem
Urticaria	Hives, a skin rash caused by allergy

Useful addresses

UNITED KINGDOM

Action Against Allergy
PO Box 278
Twickenham
TW1 4QQ
(Please send SAE)

Airedale Allergy Centre
High Hall
Steeton
Keighley
W Yorks BD20 6SB
Tel 01535 656013

Allergy Research Foundation
The Middlesex Hospital
Mortimer Street
London W1N 8AA

The Anaphylaxis Campaign
PO Box 149
Fleet
Hants GU13 9XU
Tel 01252 318723

Association of Allergen Avoidance Products and Services
Sir John Lyon House
5 High Timber Street
Upper Thames Street
London EC4V 3PA
Tel 0171 329 0950
(All products have been clinically trialled)

British Acupuncture Council
Park House
206–208 Latimer Road
London W10 6RE
Tel 0181 964 0222

British Allergy Foundation
Deepdene House
30 Bellegrove Road
Welling
Kent DA16 3BY
Tel 0181 303 8525
Helpline: 0181 303 8583

British Complementary Medicine Association
9 Soar Lane
Leicester LE3 5DE
Tel 01162 425406

British Holistic Medical Association
Rowland Thames House
Royal Shrewsbury Hospital
South

Shrewsbury SY3 8XF
Tel 01743 261155

British Homoeopathic Association
27A Devonshire Street
London W1N 1RJ
Tel 0171 935 2163

British Nutrition Foundation
High Holborn House
52–54 High Holborn
London WC1V 6RQ
Tel 0171 404 6504

Chi Centre
No 10
Greycoat Place
London SW1P 1SP
Tel 0171 222 1888
(A helpline is also available on this number)

Hale Clinic
7 Park Crescent
London W1N 3HE
Tel 0171 631 0156
(A wide variety of alternative practitioners specializing in allergy and intolerance)

Holistic Association of Reflexologists
92 Sheering Road
Old Harlow
Essex CM17 OJW
Tel 01278 429060

Institute for Complementary Medicine
PO Box 194
London SE16 1QZ
Tel 0171 237 5165

International Federation of Reflexology
76–78 Edridge Road
Croydon
Surrey CR0 1EF
Tel 0181 667 9458

International Society of Professional Aromatherapists
Ispa House
82 Ashby Road
Hinckley
Leics LE10 1SN
Tel 01455 637987

The Low Allergen House
4 Hartfield Close
Kentshill
Milton Keynes
Bucks MK7 6HN
Tel 01908 200552
(Entirely built and equipped with low-allergen products)

National Asthma Campaign
Providence House
Providence Place
London N1 0NT
Tel 0171 226 2260
Helpline 0345 01 02 03

National Eczema Society
163 Eversholt Street
London NW1 1BU
Tel 0171 388 4097

Research Council for Complementary Medicine
60 Great Ormond Street
London WC1N 3JF
Tel 0171 833 8897

**Society for the Promotion of
Nutritional Therapy**
PO Box 47
Heathfield
East Sussex TN21 8ZX
Tel 01435 867007

UCB Institute of Allergy
Star House
69 Clarendon Road
Watford
Herts WD1 1DJ

and

Chemin du Foriest
B-1420 Braine-l'Alleud
Belgium

NORTH AMERICA

**American Aromatherapy
Association**
PO Box 3679
South Pasadena
California 91031
Tel 818 457 1742

**American Holistic Medicine
Association**
4101 Lake Boone Trail
Suite 201
Raleigh
North Carolina 26707
Tel 919 787 5181

**American Naturopathic
Medicine Association**
PO Box 19221
Las Vegas
Nevada 89132
Tel 702 796 9067

**The Asthma & Allergy
Foundation of America**
1125 15th Street
NW Sta 503
Washington DC 20005

**Eczema Association for Science
and Education**
1221 South West Yamhill
Suite 303
Portland
OR 97205
Tel 503 228 4430

**The Food Allergy
Network**
10400 Eaton Place
Suite 107
Fairfax
VA 22030–2208

**National Center for
Homeopathy**
801 North Fairfax Street
Suite 306
Alexandria
VA 22314
Tel 703–548 7790

**Parents of Allergic/Asthmatic
Children (Canada)**
4007 Aspen Drive West
Edmonton
Alberta T6J 2B5

or

PO Box 4500
Edmonton
Alberta T8E 6K2

AUSTRALASIA

**Australian Association of
Asthma Foundations**
101 Princess Street
Kew
Victoria
Australia 3101
Tel: 039 853 5666

**Australian Federation for
Homeopathy**
PO Box 806
Spit Junction
New South Wales 2088

**Australian Natural Therapists
Association**
PO Box 308
Melrose Park
South Australia 5039
Tel 618 371 3222

Eczema Association of Australia
PO Box 1748 DC
Cleveland 4163
Tel 073 821 3297

National Asthma Campaign
Level One
1 Palmerston Crescent
South Melbourne
Victoria 3205
Tel 039 214 1414

APPENDIX C

Useful further reading

Allergy: A practical guide to coping, Jonathan Maberley and Honor Anthony (Crowood, UK, 1989)

Aromatherapy: An A–Z, Patricia Davis (The C W Daniel Co, UK 1992)

Food combining for health, Doris Grant and Jean Joice (Thorsons, UK, 1991).

Reflexology, Inge Dougans and Suzanne Ellis (Element, UK, 1996)

Self hypnosis, Elaine Sheehan (Element, UK, 1995)

The allergy handbook, Keith Mumby (Thorsons, UK, 1993)

The allergy survival guide, Jane Houlton (Leopard, UK, 1995)

The Elimination Diet Cookbook, Jill Carter and Alison Edwards (Element, UK, 1997)

The Rotation Diet Cookbook, Jill Carter and Alison Edwards (Element, UK, 1997)

Index

acupressure 67, 69, 72, 74

acupuncture 57, 59, 61–4, 67, 71–6, 110, 111, 116

additive(s) 15, 29, 104, 106

affirmation, positive 44, 98

Alexander technique 101

allergen(s) 3, 4, 8–15, 20, 21, 22, 23, 26

anaphylaxis, -actic 5, 6, 11, 18, 28, 40, 48, 51, 53, 77

animals 21, 25, 39

antibiotic(s) 7, 30, 42, 52, 113

antibody, -ies 3, 17, 47, 48, 53

anxiety 2, 8, 43, 44, 57, 83, 91, 92, 95, 96, 97, 103

aromatherapy 61, 85–6

asthma 1, 2, 4, 6, 9, 10, 11, 12, 14, 21, 22, 24, 41, 42, 48, 49, 51, 63, 71, 72, 75, 86, 90, 92, 97, 101, 103, 109, 117

atopy, -ic 4, 9–16, 21, 22, 25, 26, 35–41, 49, 74

autogenic training 94

babies and small children 11, 15, 16, 26, 27, 40–1, 42, 52, 74, 81, 88

biofeedback 94

blood testing 47

breathing 18, 21, 25, 26, 47, 51, 90, 91, 103, 111

Buteyko 67, 89–90

cause(s) 20, 31, 32

challenge test, 34, 35, 106, 107

chi, qi 59, 67, 69–74

Chinese herbs 11, 61, 68–74 medicine 57, 59, 67, 68, 87

choosing a practitioner 115ff

cigarette smoke 14, 21, 26, 43

clinical ecology 112 therapies 19, 66, 71, 76, 80, 86, 100

conjunctivitis 6, 10, 13, 14

contact allergy, -ies 5, 16, 20, 26–7

counselling 61, 95

cranial osteopathy 11, 67, 81–4

depression 19, 44, 64, 92, 93, 96–100

desensitization 53, 54, 76–7, 113

detoxification 113

diet, dietary 7, 18, 34, 41, 53, 73, 104, 105, 112 rotation 40, 107

drug(s) 5, 20, 29, 42, 49, 51, 52, 56, 58, 69, 79, 100

dust 3, 10, 13–15, 20–5, 36–7, 38, 47

eczema (atopic dermatitis) 1, 4, 9–11, 15, 16, 26, 43, 46, 49–53,

66, 68, 71, 74, 80, 89, 97,
109–10, 117

eggs 1, 2, 15, 18, 28, 77

elimination/exclusion diet 34,
35, 47, 77, 92, 106, 112

emotion(s) 11, 18, 19, 44, 56, 59,
66, 76, 80, 81, 83, 84, 92, 93, 95,
100, 101, 110

environment 2, 7, 23–5, 35, 39, 41,
112–13

enzyme(s) 6, 54

enzyme-potentiated
desensitization 54, 113

essential oils 56, 85, 86

evening primrose oil 109, 110

flotation therapy 94

flower remedies 100, 101

food allergies 15, 21, 27, 51, 53,
66, 71
intolerance(s) 1, 10, 12, 15, 17,
18, 112

foods, problem 28, 40, 62, 92, 105,
107, 113

food(s) 3, 10, 17, 20, 33, 34

fumes 13, 14, 21, 29, 38, 77

gastrointestinal 3, 4, 17, 33

Hay, William: Hay diet 107–8, 111

hay fever (allergic rhinitis) 1, 4,
9–15, 22, 24, 43, 48–53, 63, 66,
71, 75, 76, 97, 111

headaches 13, 72, 80, 81, 87

herbal, -ism 42, 56, 64, 67, 73, 79,
80, 89, 110, 112

histamine(s) 3, 4, 6, 13, 16, 50

history taking 45, 47, 76, 81, 105

hives (urticaria) 1, 5, 17, 50

holistic 8, 58, 59, 63, 66, 87

home, healthy 36

homeopathy, -ic 57, 63, 64, 67,
75–7, 110, 113, 114, 116

house dust mite 13, 21, 24, 25, 36,
47, 112

hydrotherapy 67, 87, 89, 110, 111

hyperactivity in children 6, 29,
97, 104

hyperventilation 90–1

hypnosis 44, 57, 63, 64, 94, 97, 99

hypnotherapy 99

immune system 2–4, 8, 10, 13,
31, 42, 54, 81, 85, 90, 97, 104,
109, 113

immunoglobulin E (IgE) 3, 4, 13,
15, 47

inflammation 7, 14, 17, 26, 49, 76,
77, 80, 109, 112

inhale(d) (substance(s)) 15, 17,
22, 23

injection immunotherapy 53

lifestyle(s) 41, 42, 43, 59, 76, 77,
78, 105

'masking' 18, 32

massage 56, 59, 67, 72, 74,
84–7, 89

mast cell(s) 3, 13, 49

medical treatment(s) 48

meditation 44, 59, 63, 99, 100,
102, 103

meridian(s) (channels) 67, 69, 71,
72, 74

migraine(s) 7, 56, 64, 105

milk, milk products 7, 28, 41, 68,
69, 77

Miller technique 54

moxibustion 71

natural medicine 59, 64, 110,
116, 117

therapies, -ist 55, 56, 58, 59, 60,
66, 114, 116

naturopathy, -path(s) 7, 73, 87, 110, 111
nettlerash (urticaria) 5, 17
neurolinguistic programming 96
neutralization injection(s) 54
nutritional therapy, -ists 7, 104, 106, 111

osteopathy 67, 80–1, 110

penicillin 20, 29
particle(s) 15, 22, 24, 31, 38
peanuts 1, 5, 28, 55
pet(s) 25, 27, 33, 37
placebo 63, 75, 100
plants causing hayfever 22–3, 27, 37
pollen 1, 3, 14, 20, 22, 38, 46, 49, 108, 112
pollen count(s) 13, 21, 39
pollution, pollutants 13, 24, 77, 112, 113
preventer(s) 49
psychotherapy 95, 96

qi, chi 59, 67
qualifications of practitioners 60, 61, 65, 117, 119
questions for self-help 32

rash(es) 3, 12, 18, 21, 25, 26, 51, 105
RAST test 34, 47
reflexology 67, 86–7
relaxation (technique(s)) 61, 77, 80, 83–5, 88, 89, 93, 94, 100, 103, 111
reliever(s) 49, 50
respiratory 4, 12, 14, 24, 33, 84, 101

rhinitis 6, 10, 12, 13, 21, 22, 24, 49, 50

sensitivity, -ies 6, 7, 10, 26, 29, 45, 47, 48, 104
sensitization 3, 10, 11, 13, 14, 16, 22, 25, 28, 41, 52, 77, 107
Shiatsu 67, 74
skin 1, 4, 16–18, 26, 39, 46, 51, 52, 54, 69, 74, 79, 83, 87, 89, 98, 112
skin prick testing 46
smoke, smoking 10, 26, 29, 37, 42
stings 17, 51, 54, 80, 97
stress 15, 19, 26, 41, 43, 57, 61, 64, 68, 74, 77–9, 85, 86, 91, 93, 95–103, 112
substance(s) 20, 22, 22, 26–7, 33, 34, 38, 40, 43, 45, 47, 48, 60, 75, 76, 92, 104, 111, 112
swelling 3, 5, 11, 12, 13, 17, 46, 49, 51, 68
symptoms 1, 6, 8

testing, self- 33, 35
   professional 34, 45
training of practitioners 117, 119

urticaria (hives or nettlerash) 1, 5, 17, 18, 49, 50, 69

vaccine(s) 54, 55
visualization 97
vitamins 108, 111

working environment 7, 39
workplace 14, 26

yin and yang 59, 67, 68, 73
yoga 72, 102, 103

BHMA Tapes for Health

*Practical self-help packages designed by
experts to make taking care of yourself easier*

Imagery For Relaxation by Duncan Johnson

Exercises in visualization to help relaxation and influence the functions of the body and mind. To provide yourself with the opportunity to learn more about your attitudes and neglected needs. To harness the forces of the creative mind and change negative attitudes to life.

Getting To Sleep by Ashley Conway

A practical help with insomnia. Promotes relaxation and positive thinking to put you in touch with your body's 'normal' sleep pattern.

Introduction To Meditation by Dr Sarah Eagger

This tape is a progressive learning programme of meditation exercises. Teaching you how to begin using meditation for increasing your peace of mind and well-being.

Coping With Persistent Pain by Dr James Hawkins

Teaches relaxation skills in a greater depth, and how to apply those skills as a coping method during daily activities. To help promote some form of normality into a life of constant pain.

Coping With Stress by Dr David Peters

A programme to teach you how to build the relaxation response into your life. Understanding stress and dealing with it through relaxation techniques.

The Breath Of Life by Dr Patrick Pietroni

A muscular relaxation technique which explores the connection between stress and our breathing rhythm. With exercises on how to control breathing to alleviate symptoms of stress.

Please write to the British Holistic Medical Association at Rowland Thomas House, Royal Shrewsbury Hospital South, Shrewsbury, Shropshire, SY3 8XF for full details of tapes and mail order service.